Procedures in Diagnostic Radiology

Procedures in Diagnostic Radiology

Terence Doyle MD, FRACR
Professor of Radiology
University of Otago, Dunedin
New Zealand

William S C Hare MD, FRACR
Professor of Radiology
The University of Melbourne
The Royal Melbourne Hospital, Victoria
Australia

Kenneth Thomson MB ChB, FRACR
Associate, Department of Radiology
The University of Melbourne
The Royal Melbourne Hospital, Victoria
Australia

Brian Tress MB BS, FRACR
First Assistant, Department of Radiology
The University of Melbourne
The Royal Melbourne Hospital, Victoria
Australia

CHURCHILL LIVINGSTONE
EDINBURGH LONDON MELBOURNE AND NEW YORK 1989

CHURCHILL LIVINGSTONE
Medical Division of Longman Group UK Limited

Distributed in the United States of America by
Churchill Livingstone Inc., 1560 Broadway, New
York, N.Y. 10036, and by associated companies,
branches and representatives throughout the world.

First published 1989

ISBN 0 443 02982 2

British Library Cataloguing in Publication Data
Procedures in diagnostic radiology.
   1. Medicine. Radiology
   I. Doyle, Terence
   616.07'57

Library of Congress Cataloging in Publication Data
Procedures in diagnostic radiology/Terence Doyle . . . [et al.].
      p.   cm.
   Includes index.
   1. Diagnosis, Radioscopic.   I. Doyle, Terence.
   [DNLM: 1. Radiography — methods.   WN 200 P963]
RC78.P84 1989
616.07'57 — dc 19

Produced by Longman Singapore Publishers (Pte) Ltd.
Printed in Singapore.

Preface

This book is intended to be a reference work for radiology trainees learning to do practical procedures for the first time and also for practitioners called upon to perform such procedures when they may be outside their usual range of experience.

The authors are all working radiologists with a collectively wide experience in diagnostic and interventional studies. The book therefore has a heavily practical emphasis, considering not only the standard ways of performing the procedures but also how to overcome the problems and difficulties likely to be encountered.

Dunedin, New Zealand   T.D.

Contents

1

Introduction

ASSESSMENT OF PATIENTS

Before any patient is 'imaged', in an ideal situation they should be assessed by a member of the radiology department who is able to make decisions relating to the timing and type of procedure required to make the diagnosis with the least risk, at the least cost to the patient and to the community.

For instance it is not cost-effective to subject a patient with suspected acromegaly to a battery of radiological investigations from heel pad thickness to computed tomography to simply confirm the diagnosis if it has been made by growth hormone assay.

If a female of child-bearing age thinks there is a possibility that she may be pregnant then any examination involving ionizing radiation exposure to the pelvis should be postponed until her menstrual period starts unless there is a pressing medical indication for the examination.

A history of exposure to hepatitis 'B' is very important particularly if arteriography or other invasive examinations are planned. In cases of doubt the patient should be screened for antigens and the examination postponed until results are available. If antigens are present then special protective measures will be undertaken during the examination.

Patients with severe heart, renal or liver disease may be unable to survive invasive examinations unless they are modified to accommodate the limitations imposed by their disease. In particular patients with myeloma undergoing contrast examinations should not be dehydrated because of the risk of acute renal failure. The rigorous bowel preparation performed in preparation for a double contrast barium enema may be dangerous in a patient with ulcerative colitis.

In actual practice referring physicians may not commonly accept kindly the opinion of a radiologist regarding the timing of, or the need for, investigation of their patient. Radiological examinations are in most centres still 'ordered' rather than 'requested'. The clinical information provided is often inadequate.

Because of the rapid increase in imaging technology the radiologist is often the only person who is in a position to provide a logical and cost-

1

effective plan of investigation. This can be done by ensuring that all imaging 'request forms' are approved by the radiologist in charge of the area in which the investigation will be performed. If it is to be done properly the previous imaging examinations and often the case record notes must be perused. This is the practice in the Royal Melbourne only for selected examinations which are 'high cost' such as computed tomography or 'high risk' such as interventional angiography.

Simple examinations of the chest or limbs are of sufficiently high volume to render any pre-examination vetting impractical and sometimes the films are not seen by a radiologist before the patient departs.

The films from each examination should be viewed by a radiologist, and compared with previous examinations if possible, as they emerge from the film processor.

Contraindications to imaging procedures depends largely on the patients and their disease. Uterine angiography for instance is not recommended in early pregnancy but other decisions are less easy to make. Is carotid arteriography to confirm satisfactory clipping of a cerebral aneurysm necessary? If the result of the imaging examination will not influence the treatment or course of a disease process is the examination justified?

Absolute contraindications for examinations without the risk of ionizing radiation or the risk of contrast media are few. A history of severe reaction to contrast or the combination of dehydration and myeloma are relative contraindications to vascular contrast media. In most cases the examination can be modified or the patient's circumstances be changed by treatment to allow the disease process to be imaged adequately.

The particular indications and contraindications for each procedure are listed in the text.

SEDATION FOR DIAGNOSTIC PROCEDURES

If the procedure is not painful and the radiologist or X-ray technician explains what is required then sedation is not indicated or desirable. The worst part of most radiology procedures is the uninformed imagination of an anxious patient. Since patients are grouped by unit the chances are that the patient in the next bed can provide a horrific description of the procedure and its complications.

The anxious patient is conveniently premedicated with oral diazepam 10 mg 2 hours prior to the procedure. The diazepam appears to give the patient a shortened perception of the passage of time in addition to reducing anxiety.

It is not sensible to place a nervous patient outside an examination room from which are emanating a series of shrieks and moans from a patient in pain.

A combination of opiate and atropine is used as a premedication but the patient is often nauseated by this combination and the addition of metoclopramide (Maxolon) may be required. In our experience a nervous and uncooperative patient may become uncontrollable and move unpredictably when stimulated while heavily sedated.

When the procedure is painful at the point of insertion of a needle then a large volume of low strength local anaesthetic is often more effective than sedation. This works well in nephrostomies but is not suitable for external carotid embolization. If severe pain is to be expected or the procedure will be unbearably long then neuroleptanaesthesia, epidural anaesthesia or a general anaesthetic is indicated.

Post-procedural pain relief may be required after minor examinations and is always required after renal embolization due to the infarct produced. After-care of radiology procedures, particularly the invasive ones, is the radiologist's responsibility.

EMERGENCIES IN THE RADIOLOGY DEPARTMENT

Prophylaxis

Emergencies in the radiology department are usually medical. As some patients are more likely than others to cause an emergency then these 'high risk' patients should be under observation by a nurse, X-ray technician or doctor for the duration of their examination and they should be accompanied to and from the department if necessary with a cardiac monitor and by a person who is familiar with the patient's medical problem.

On arrival in the department the patient case record should be checked for a history of allergy, diseases such as phaeochromocytoma and myeloma, and if steroids have been given recently in significant doses.

If the examination is likely to precipitate an emergency then there should be resuscitation equipment in the room ready for immediate use. If the patient is in a parlous state the examination should be performed only if it is essential to the immediate management.

Although modern X-ray equipment is earthed and safe in an anaesthetic room, some older equipment cannot be made completely safe with respect to earth current leakage and is not suitable for use in the presence of an explosive anaesthetic gas. Such machines should be clearly labelled or preferably replaced.

Patients who have a documented history of a bronchospasm, circulatory collapse, or cardiac arryhthmia following contrast injection should be assessed by the radiologist and, if indicated, the examination postponed until pre-testing and prophylactic regime of corticosteriods undertaken. The non-ionic contrasts appear to offer much greater safety with regard to 'allergy' and are now indicated in all cases of previous reaction to contrast.

It is essential that all staff in the radiology department, including the non-medical personnel, are trained and practised in cardiopulmonary resuscitation and know where the emergency equipment is kept. As emergencies are for the most part unexpected and infrequent, the staff may become complacent and unready. In The Royal Melbourne Hospital the Coronary Intensive Care Unit 'arrest team' attends all emergencies in the radiology department. This overcomes any inexperience through lack of practice on the part of the radiology staff and speeds the transfer of the patient to Intensive Care if required.

In cases of contrast 'allergy' there is now evidence that an intravenous challenge injection will be of prognostic value if a rigorous protocol is followed in which sufficient time is allowed after each test injection for a reaction to develop. If a severe reaction does occur after a test dose, the need for contrast examination should be carefully reassessed and non-ionic contrast (Iopamiro) or a corticosteroid premedication used.

Whenever contrast is given it is prudent to use a needle set which can be left in position until the end of the procedure in case a contrast reaction occurs. Onset of contrast reactions have been reported several hours after injection.

TREATMENT

Contrast media reactions

These are probably the most common emergencies in a radiology department and most occur in the urography area (Lalli 1980). If a contrast reaction should occur during an excretion urogram and the patient's condition permits, at least one roentgenogram should be made of the renal area as it may be diagnostic and it is likely that the examination will not be repeated.

Reactions are conveniently divided into three groups; minor, vaso-vagal and major.

Minor reactions

A minor reaction is usually evidenced by the presence of hives or an erythematous skin rash. The patient is often unaware of the rash and in such cases treatment is hardly necessary. If the patient complains of itching then intramuscular anti-histamines are given as a single dose.

Nausea and vomiting may occur after even a small amount of contrast and even if no treatment is given may not occur after much larger doses for a film run. If nausea is persistent then an anti-emetic (metoclopramide) is given intravenously. Vomiting after injections for urography is more common than with either injections for intravenous digital subtraction angiography or for arteriography. The reasons for this are not clear.

Vaso-vagal reactions

A feeling of impending doom accompanied by pallor and slow pulse indicate a vaso-vagal reaction which is likely to be due to fear or the radiologist's attitude. Patient anxiety is thought by some to be the sole cause of 'contrast reactions' (Shehadi & Toniolo 1980) and if the patient is nervous then premedication with diazepam, a narcotic, and atropine is likely to produce a smooth examination. Many of the 'contrast reactions' in the patient history appear on close examination to be vaso-vagal in nature.

Major reactions

Major reactions are those in which the patient experiences bronchospasm, circulatory collapse or loss of consciousness. The treatment of such conditions is the intravenous injection of 1:10 000 adrenaline in 1 ml aliquots as required, and supportive methods aimed at maintaining an adequate airway and cardiac output. Cardiopulmonary resuscitation may be necessary.

Corticosteroids are usually administered but the rationale for this in the acute situation is unclear as their effects are not active immediately. Antihistamines are also usually given but after adrenaline the sense of this could also be questioned. Epsilon-amino-caproic acid may also have a protective effect. The patient is then transferred to the intensive care area for the next 24 hours as a further delayed reaction may occur.

Other medical emergencies

In a hospital environment there is always the possibility that a patient will suffer a cardiac arrest, pulmonary embolus, stroke or other event which is unrelated to the examination.

The first person on the scene should call for help, (preferably by way of a 'cardiac arrest alarm button') and immediately ensure that the airway is clear. If the patient has stopped breathing begin mouth to mouth respiration as an annoxic arrested heart will often resume beating normally when ventilation is adequate. (The chance of contracting AIDS or other infectious diseases this way is very slight.) If the airway cannot be cleared from above a 'tracheostomy' can be performed by passage of a large bore needle directly into the trachea below the cricoid.

Next evaluate the cardiac status. If in doubt start cardiac compression by alternating three or four compressions for each ventilation. If a second person has arrived one should ventilate while the other performs cardiac compression. A compression rate of about 60 per minute is sufficient. A higher rate is very tiring.

The arrival of the 'arrest team' will provide a defibrillator, ECG, and the drugs necessary to treat any arryhthmia and electrolyte imbalance. An endotracheal tube should be inserted and artificial ventilation with oxygen started if the patient is still not breathing spontaneously.

Access to the circulation may be obtained via the arm veins or by the femoral veins. There is usually insufficient time for a cut-down and small veins are not likely to provide good central access for drugs, especially if the vein is distal and the cardiac output is poor.

If a satisfactory heart rate and blood pressure are maintained then the ventilation should be continued. If after 10 minutes or so, with adequate ventilation and cardiac compression, the patient is still non-responsive without heart beat, blood pressure or respiration then the resuscitation attempt should be abandoned. It is often harder to stop resuscitation than to start it.

REFERENCES

Lalli A F 1980 Contrast media reactions: data analysis and hypothesis. Radiology 137: 869
Shehadi W H, Toniolo G 1980 Adverse reactions to contrast media (Report from the Committee on Safety of Contrast Media of the International Society of Radiology). Radiology 137: 299–302

2

Urinary tract

INTRAVENOUS PYELOGRAPHY

Indications

1. The basic method for displaying the anatomy of the kidneys, upper urinary tract and bladder.
2. Used to detect functional abnormalities, e.g. resulting from ureteric obstruction, or associated with renal artery stenosis.

Equipment

The intravenous injection

1. Butterfly needle, gauge 19 or 21.
2. Contrast medium. Water soluble ionic or non-ionic medium according to patients' risk category. (See 'Difficulties and complications'.) Approximately 20 g of iodine for adults. With ionic media meglumine salts are preferred because of lower toxicity even though sodium salts have been shown to give slightly higher iodine concentration in urine.
3. Resuscitation equipment for severe contrast reactions. In particular, an airway, a means of administering air or oxygen, a knowledge of cardiac massage and drugs including adrenaline 1 : 10 000.

Radiographic equipment

1. Tomographic facility an essential requirement.
2. Low kV techniques (i.e. 60 kV or less) required to enhance contrast. High mA necessary to keep exposure times as short as possible.
3. Abdominal compression belt (separate from ureteric compression) attached to table to steady patient and reduce abdominal thickness to shorten exposure times (Fig. 2.1).
4. Inflatable ureteric compression belt, attached to patient, but not to table, with quick release mechanism. Preferably separate balloons for each ureter (Fig. 2.1).
5. Bucky, screen–film–cassette combination.

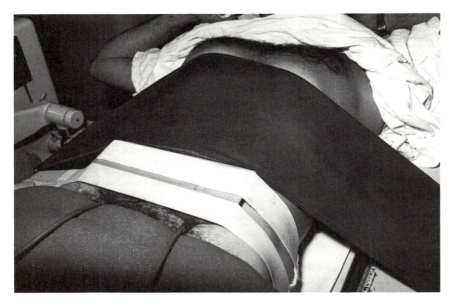

Fig. 2.1 Arrangement of compression bands during intravenous pyelography. The broad upper belt, fixed to the table, steadies the patient and reduces the thickness of the abdomen. The lower ureteric compression belt, attached to the patient only, has two separate inflatable bags to compress each ureter.

Patient preparation

1. No fluid or food restriction. The patient is advised to eat and drink normally. Fluid restriction increases the risk of renal impairment following contrast injection particularly in diabetics with chronic renal failure. Following examination the patient is encouraged to maintain a high fluid intake for 24 hours.
2. Mild laxative on evening before examination.
3. Question about previous contrast reactions and relevant history, e.g. analgesic intake, diabetes, etc. If a previous severe contrast reaction use non-ionic contrast medium.
4. Empty bladder. Immediately prior to examination. Use catheter if necessary.

Technique

1. To avoid missing small opaque calculi or calcified foci, it is essential that adequate plain radiographs are obtained prior to contrast injection. Oblique views, tomography, and views on inspiration and expiration may be required. Plain films must be carefully inspected before contrast injection and further views made if in doubt. Calculi are not infrequently overlooked.

2. Although some films in the series should include kidneys, ureter and bladder the majority of views should be coned to particular areas of interest for greater detail.
3. Injection of the contrast medium.
   (a) Although arguable a reasonable practice is to inject 5 ml of contrast and to wait a few minutes to see if a major reaction occurs. The time can be spent in questioning the patient concerning relevant matters such as analgesic intake, i.e. essential knowledge when interpreting abnormal pyelograms.
   (b) The remainder of contrast is injected rapidly as a bolus taking about one minute and a renal film, preferably a tomogram, is made immediately to show the nephrographic phase.
4. In all cases, except suspected reno-vascular hypertension (see p. 10), the usual procedure is to make coned renal films:
   (a) Five minutes from conclusion of injection without ureteric compression. Apply ureteric compression (Fig. 2.1).
   (b) A renal film at 10 minutes from injection with compression applied.
5. Urography requires continual supervision by the radiologist. Careful assessment at the 10 minute mark of the films obtained determines the programme of views to complete the examination. The series will usually include:
   (a) A full length film of the filled ureters immediately after release of compression.
   (b) Coned views of the filled bladder including obliques if pathology suspected.
   (c) A film immediately after micturition to include the entire tract.
The following comments may be helpful if elucidating particular problems.

Apparent unilateral non-function of the kidney

1. If a nephrogram was demonstrated but no outlining of the pelvicalyceal system, ureteric obstruction is likely, particularly if the kidney appears swollen. A further loading dose of contrast medium (equal to the original injection) and delayed filming after several hours or more may demonstrate the obstructed ureter.
2. Availability of ultrasound allows immediate detection of pelvicalyceal dilatation. If so, antegrade pyelography (see later) can be performed as an immediate follow-on procedure.

Suspected calculi

1. Comprehensive plain films are essential particularly in all patients with pain.
2. When a filling defect in contrast films is detected due to a low density

calculus, blood clot, tumour or sloughed papilla, study the plain films of the site very carefully, and if unclear repeat the plain film on another occasion. A faint opacity, indicating a stone, may be detected in retrospect.

3. The after release film should clarify the position of small opacities in the line of the ureter. If not, the ureteric compression should be reapplied and a further contrast injection, if necessary, given. Further views, including obliques, after the second release of ureteric compression should clarify the situation. Only rarely should retrograde ureteric catheterization be needed to determine whether an opacity is in or outside a ureter. The radiologist should look on such a requirement as a failure of his IVP technique.

Prostatism

1. In frail, very elderly men the essential information from pyelography can be elicited with no special patient preparation and a minimum of effort.
2. Plain films of the urinary tract will exclude obvious calculi, and reveal prostatic bone metastases.
3. A full length view after contrast will show back pressure dilatation of the ureters, will provide some idea of renal size and function, and show trabeculation, diverticula and evidence of bladder tumour.
4. A view of the bladder base on a 25 × 20 cm film provides the best view for assessing the intravesical extension of the prostate. The centre ray is angled 12° cranially and is centred to the inferior margin of the symphysis pubis.
5. A full length film after micturition provides an assessment of residual urine.

Lasix washout test in suspected pelvi-ureteric junction (PUJ) obstruction

1. When an after micturition film on intravenous pyelography shows a degree of retention and distension suggesting PUJ obstruction, some assessment of the degree of obstruction can be made by repeating the contrast injection with 20 mg of Lasix.
2. Films made at 10-minute intervals allow comparison with the other kidney. The degree of additional distension after Lasix compared with the normal side, is an index of the degree of obstruction.

Suspected reno-vascular hypertension

The examination aims to show functional differences between the two kidneys. The ischaemic kidney is smaller and contrast appears later. Also, because the ischaemic kidney excretes a smaller urine volume and reabsorbs more sodium, the ischaemic pyelogram is denser.

1. After rapid bolus injection of contrast, films of the kidneys are made at 1, 2, 5 and 9 minutes without ureteric compression. This allows assessment of appearance time, and measurement of renal sizes.
2. Ureteric compression is applied and a further renal view is made at 15 minutes. This may show increased contrast density on the ischaemic side.
3. Further views if necessary are then prescribed depending on the appearances obtained. If the findings suggest unilateral ischaemia, a view 5 minutes after 20 mg Lasix may show delayed washout on the ischaemic side.

Remember if focal disease, e.g. scarring of reflux nephropathy is present, the assessment of renal ischaemia by IVP is unreliable, as it depends on the parenchyma of the normal and ischaemic kidney being morphologically normal.

Difficulties and complications of IVP

Contrast medium reactions

Over 20% of patients experience some reaction following the intravenous injection. The majority are trivial including nausea and minor urticaria. A few patients are more severely affected with hypotension and degrees of circulatory collapse or bronchospasm. A major collapse with asystole accounts for most of the reported mortality ranging from 1 : 40 000 to 1 : 117 000 IVP examinations (Ansell 1976). Such a reaction usually occurs in the five minutes following injection and 90% of severe reactions occur within 15 minutes. The patient must not be left unattended during this period.

A drill should be established and practised to deal with catastrophic circulatory collapse. If an adequate cardio-respiratory status can be maintained during the crucial period prior to admission to an intensive care facility the prognosis should be good.

For minor reactions intravenous antihistamine preparations are usually effective. Minor degrees of bronchospasm are overcome with subcutaneous adrenaline 1 : 10 000.

For a major collapse the team involved should take the following steps:
1. Insert an oral airway to immobilize the tongue.
2. Commence cardiac massage and continue uninterrupted.
3. Provide room air or oxygen under pressure using a face mask. The Oxyviva type apparatus is simple and effective (Fig. 2.2).
4. Intravenous adrenaline 1 : 10 000 may be given in doses of 1 ml/min up to a total of 5 ml. With the availability of intensive care facilities and ECG monitoring, additional steps may be taken including bicarbonate infusion, endotracheal airway, cardiac defibrillation and intravenous corticosteroids.

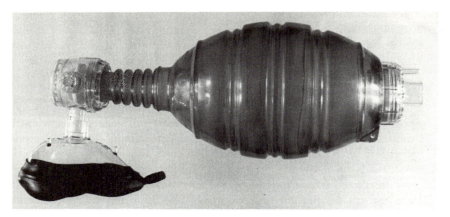

Fig. 2.2 The Oxy-viva apparatus for delivering room air to the patient by manual compression of the bag.

The motto is 'be prepared'. The outcome of a major reaction is largely dependent on the expertise of those in the IVP room conducting the procedure. Regular practice of the emergency drill is advisable.

Prevention. Patients at higher risk of experiencing iodine contrast reaction include those who experienced a previous severe reaction, elderly patients particularly with compromised cardiac or renal function, diabetics, asthmatics and those with an allergic history. Use of non-ionic or low osmolar media, e.g. iopamidol, iohexol or ioxaglate, is recommended for intravenous pyelography in those patients because of the demonstrated lower reaction rate and incidence of severe reactions. Recently it has been shown that the very low reaction rate of non-ionic media, which are very expensive, can be matched by using ionic media with corticosteroid cover (Lasser et al 1987). One 32 mg tablet of methylprednisolone is taken on the evening before examination and a second tablet on the morning of examination at least 2 hours before the contrast injection. This regime of steroid cover is recommended for all previous severe reactions.

Arm vein thrombosis

Stagnation of large volumes of hyperosmolar contrast in the arm veins may cause thrombosis. After injection the arm should be exercised briefly to disperse residual contrast. The butterfly needle should be placed away from the elbow flexure for this purpose.

ANTEGRADE PYELOGRAPHY

The availability of ultrasound for localization, and the atraumatic Chiba puncture needle have made percutaneous access to the pelvicalyceal system feasible. Antegrade pyelography has replaced retrograde pyelography in many situations.

Indications

1. To demonstrate the site and nature of ureteric obstruction.
2. To perform pressure/flow studies in suspected functional ureteric obstruction (Whitaker 1979).

Equipment

1. Ultrasound equipment for non-functioning kidneys.
2. Items for intravenous contrast injection to produce pyelogram in functioning kidney.
3. 23G Chiba type needle 12 cm long with stilette.

Patient preparation

Local anaesthesia.

Technique

1. Patient position. Prone and slightly flexed over a firm pillow in the epigastrium. Do not elevate head or shoulders on pillow.

2. Localizing renal pelvis. Functioning kidney. Introduce butterfly IV needle whilst patient supine. Use hand for preference to avoid dislodgement when prone. Inject IV water soluble contrast to produce pyelogram. Using intensifier to localize pelvis, mark skin for needle puncture. Avoid parallax by placing renal pelvis in centre of the intensifier field. Use ureteric compression in undilated systems.

Non-functioning kidney. Using ultrasound, in longitudinal and transverse planes, with suspended respiration, mark site of skin puncture over the renal pelvis. Measure the depth of the pelvis from skin surface.

3. Local anaesthesia. Using 10 cm needle introduce LA down to the kidney during suspended respiration. If a rib overlies the renal pelvis, the skin puncture should be made lower and the needle angled superiorly to avoid it.

4. Pelvis puncture. Pass the needle downwards percutaneously towards the renal pelvis, checking direction by image intensifier if pelvis opacified. A real time ultrasound biopsy transducer may be used but is not essential. When the needle has been passed to the determined depth the stilette is removed and connecting tube and syringe are attached to the needle. Using gentle aspiration the needle is withdrawn. Urine flow into the tubing signals entry into the pelvis (Fig. 2.3).

Note: The pelvis is often deeper than expected.

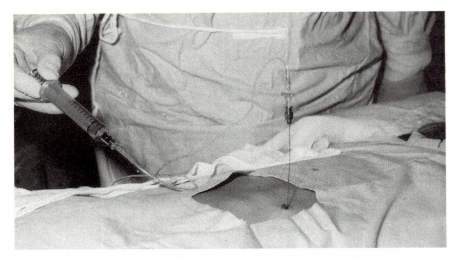

Fig. 2.3 Antegrade pyelography. With the patient prone a 23 gauge needle has been placed in the renal pelvis and urine aspirated.

5. Urine specimen. A specimen of urine is aspirated and placed in a sterile container for analysis. By holding the connector tubing vertical the hydrostatic pressure in the pelvis is measured (normal less than 20 cm of urine above the needle point).

6. Contrast injection.

(a) A few millilitres of contrast should be injected to check that the needle is accurately placed.

(b) If markedly distended the pelvicalyceal system should be aspirated before outlining with contrast medium.

(c) If after contrast replacement the point of ureteric obstruction is not clearly seen, 0.5 ml of oily medium (Pantopaque or Myodil) should be injected. After withdrawing the needle a radiograph is made with the patient erect and the oily material will show the point of hold up.

Difficulties and complications

The needle puncture, per se, is virtually free from complications.

1. Bacteraemia and septicaemia. Overdistension of an infected pelvicalyceal system may result in bloodstream infection. Aspiration prior to contrast injection will reduce this risk.

2. Urinoma. Overdistension of the pelvicalyceal system with contrast results in forniceal rupture and urine may accumulate in the retroperitoneum.

3. Haematuria. Some blood staining may occur following puncture but rarely is of any consequence.

RETROGRADE PYELOGRAPHY

Indications

1. To demonstrate the upper urinary tract in patients with diminished renal function. If ureteric obstruction is present antegrade pyelography is now preferred to retrograde pyelography.
2. To clarify findings on intravenous pyelography, e.g. whether an opacity lies in a ureter or not. Most of these problems can be solved by the intravenous method if the problem is realized at the time of examination.

Equipment

1. Standard X-ray table with Bucky diaphragm.
2. Image intensifier fluoroscope is a more sophisticated alternative and provides accurate filming.
3. Ureteral catheter connections (VPI) (hypodermic needles will do).
4. Water soluble contrast medium.

Patient preparation

Usually the patient is delivered to the department from the operating theatre with ureteric catheters in place. At the most a general anaesthetic will have been given and the patient may not be fully cooperative.

Technique

1. Adequate plain films are obtained and studied.
2. A film is made after injecting 5 ml of contrast. Both catheters can be injected simultaneously.
3. If a fluoroscope is not used, the first film must be checked for overfilling. Further injections are arranged including AP and oblique views.
4. The radiologist must know whether the catheters are to be left in or removed. If they are to be removed it may be helpful to inject during withdrawal and make a film immediately after.
5. If necessary delayed films should be obtained to check on drainage if ureteric obstruction is suspected.

Difficulties and complications

1. Ureteric perforation. Occasionally the catheter will lie outside the ureter. Careful withdrawal until the tip is in the lumen may allow the examination to proceed. No complications result.

2. Overfilling. Spasm of the ureter about the catheter results in forniceal rupture and contrast extravasation. If fluoroscopic control is not used it is important to inject only 5 ml as a maximum for the first radiograph.

3. Reflux anuria. Oliguria and even significant periods of anuria have been reported following bilateral examination. Overfilling may contribute to the incidence.

PERCUTANEOUS NEPHROSTOMY

Indications

1. To provide temporary or permanent urinary diversion.
2. To provide access to the upper urinary tract for various procedures including:
   (a) removal of urinary calculi
   (b) placement of stents
   (c) closure of fistulae
   (d) dilatation of strictures.

Equipment

1. As for antegrade pyelography.
2. A percutaneous nephrostomy set including a Chiba type needle, 0.46 mm (0.018 in) guidewire, introducing catheter with cannula, and 0.89 mm (0.035 in) J guidewire. This Cook–Cope type of set allows a nephrostomy to be made atraumatically as only a 21 gauge needle is introduced initially after which the track is dilated. Larger catheter sheathed needle sets can be used and are cheaper, but are better reserved for dilated pelves when single renal puncture can be anticipated.
3. Set of dilating catheters, e.g. Amplatz dilators (Cook) up to 30F size. These can be reused. Alternatively a balloon dilating catheter can be used (Cook) but is expensive. The balloon is sufficiently long to dilate the entire track and may be better tolerated than multiple dilating catheters.
4. Self-retaining pigtail nephrostomy catheter, e.g. Cook–Cope type, sizes 10F or 12F. For larger bore nephrostomies other catheters may be adapted. Foley catheters are suitable if an end hole is fashioned using the Pollack hole punch (Cook) to allow introduction over a guide. A coaxial arrangement of catheters may be used with the inner tube passing down the ureter.
5. A suitable nephrostomy drainage bag, e.g. Squibb Stomadhesive wafer set, or Bardek leg bag with suitable soft lightweight connector tubing.
6. A Molnar disc to secure the nephrostomy tube to the skin.

Patient preparation

1. The degree of discomfort experienced relates to the degree of nephrostomy dilatation required at the initial procedure. Sufficient sedation and

analgesia can be achieved by titrating doses of diazepam (20–30 mg) and pethidine (100–150 mg) given in diluted form through an indwelling IV butterfly needle, using separate syringes.

2. Widespread infiltration down into the renal capsule using a mixture of 20 ml of 1% xylocaine with 1 : 200 000 adrenaline, 20 ml 1% xylocaine and 20 ml N saline. The entire 60 ml may be used in adults but less is usually sufficient. A considerable volume should be allowed to diffuse in the perirenal space. Many patients can be dilated in one stage to 24F. In others dilatation must be staged over several days. In very few is general anaesthesia required.

3. Solid food intake should be curtailed for four hours before the procedure.

Technique

1. Patient lies prone over a pillow and antegrade pyelography is performed (as described previously). This serves several purposes:
   (a) Direct contrast injection assists localization with the intensifier.
   (b) Injection of dilute contrast distends the system immediately before nephrostomy puncture.
   (c) The needle in the pelvis is some help in assessing depth and angle for the oblique nephrostomy puncture.
   (d) The needle to some extent immobilizes the kidney.

2. The nephrostomy skin puncture site is selected immediately below the lowest rib in the renal angle, i.e. lateral extent of sacrospinalis. Local anaesthesia is carried down to the renal capsule. With a scalpel a puncture is made through the layers of the posterior abdominal wall and sufficiently large to take the desired nephrostomy tube.

3. The fine 21 gauge puncture needle is passed to the level of the renal capsule adjacent to the calyx to be punctured. The correct depth is checked by observing differential movement of the needle tip and the selected calyx during respiration. If the needle has greater amplitude than the calyx it lies too deep (i.e. with an under table X-ray tube) and vice versa. The calyx is then punctured under vision with the intensifier during suspended respiration. In unobstructed systems the calyx should be distended at the time by puncture by injecting dilute contrast through the needle in the renal pelvis.

4. The stilette is removed and the 0.46 mm (0.018 in) guide introduced into the pelvicalyceal system (Fig. 2.4A). The needle is removed.

5. The introducing catheter with stiffening cannula is carefully slid over the fine guidewire using a rotary action (Fig. 2.4B). As the catheter tip enters the calyx the metal cannula and guide should be gradually withdrawn until the tip of the catheter is well into the drainage system.

6. The 0.89 mm (0.035 in) J wire is now passed into the catheter and passes out a side hole which lies 1.5 cm proximal to the tip. This may

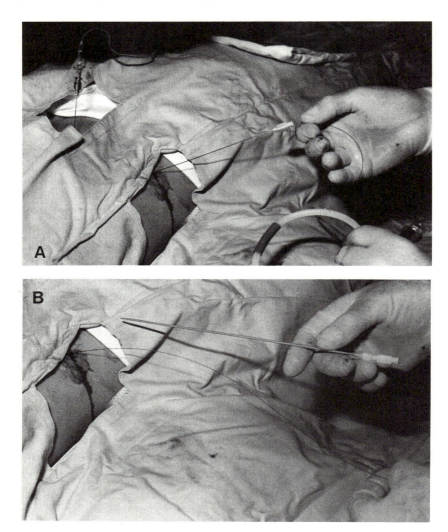

Fig. 2.4 Percutaneous nephrostomy. (A) The 0.46 mm (0.018 in) guide is being introduced through the 21 gauge needle into the pelvicalyceal system. Note the antegrade pyelography needle remains in position. (B) After removal of the needle the introducing catheter with cannula is prepared for introduction over the wire.

require some manipulation and sometimes a J wire with a tip curve radius of 1.5 mm is required, to pass out through the side hole.

7. The introducing catheter is now removed and dilators are passed over the 0.89 mm (0.035 in) guide starting at 6F. The intravenous analgesia should be reinforced. It is most satisfactory if the guidewire can be placed in the ureter. This avoids buckling during dilatation and dislodgement is less likely.

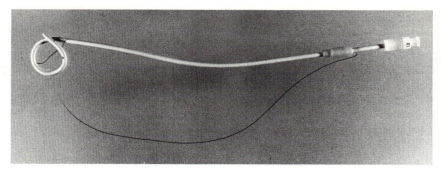

Fig. 2.5 Cook–Cope type loop nephrostomy catheter. The thread locks the loop in position avoiding extrusion.

8. Dilatation is continued to the desired calibre. A suitable sized self-retaining nephrostomy tube is then inserted (Fig. 2.5) and is clipped off or drained to a bag. The Molnar disc is used to fix the catheter to the skin and the adhesive wafer is applied to allow direct attachment of the drainage bag (Fig. 2.6).

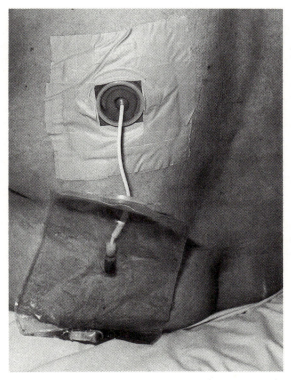

Fig. 2.6 Percutaneous nephrostomy drainage. The bag has been unclipped to show the means of fixing the catheter.

Difficulties and complications

1. Septicaemia. If infection is present in the upper urinary tract, particularly associated with ureteric obstruction, septicaemia may result and antibiotic cover is indicated in all such cases. Urine from the initial puncture should be cultured.

2. Perforation of adjacent organs. Placing the nephrostomy well laterally is more comfortable for the patient lying in bed, but carries the risk of perforating the descending colon on the left and the liver on the right. Perforating the liver has been uneventful. Penetration of the colon with the nephrostomy tube has led to pyonephrosis. Gaseous distension of the descending colon should be noted at fluoroscopy and care taken to confine the nephrostomy puncture to the renal angle. If a nephrostomy is found to pass through the colon a second nephrostomy should be performed prior to removal of the contaminated tube.

3. Damage to renal pedicle. The renal pelvis may be easily perforated medially, but with small instruments this is usually uneventful.

4. Dislodged nephrostomy tube. Straight tubes will be extruded from the upper urinary tract, and some restraining device is necessary. The Cope loop, and similar nephrostomy tubes, is excellent. It has a thread passing along the lumen which allows the loop to be firmly held in position. Such tubes should be changed every 3 months in long-term cases because of encrustation. Straight tubes can be stable if a second catheter is placed coaxially through the straight tube and particularly if the inner tube is placed well down the ureter.

PERCUTANEOUS REMOVAL OF URINARY CALCULI

In recent years new methods for dealing with stones in the upper urinary tract have been developed including endoscopic and extra-corporeal lithotripsy. Patient discomfort and length of hospital stay have been reduced with the replacement of operative surgery with less invasive methods. Radiological techniques for displacing, dissolving, disintegrating and extracting stones have evolved which contribute to the management of these patients either by the radiologist alone, or in association with the urologist. This chapter is devoted to procedures which logically are the role of the radiologist in management of renal and ureteric stones.

Renal stones

The radiologist may be required:
1. To perform percutaneous nephrostomy prior to endoscopic stone removal and ultrasonic lithotripsy. The technique is described in a previous section, but the following points apply to these cases:
   (a) The site of entry to the pelvicalyceal system must be accurate. Care

should be taken to enter the calyx lateral and not medial to the site of a calyceal stone.

(b) For staghorn calculi occupying most of the space of the pelvis, maximal distention should be achieved at the time of nephrostomy needle puncture by using ureteric compression and saline injection through the previously placed antegrade pyelography needle.

2. To insert irrigating catheters as a preliminary to dissolving uric acid, cystine, and some infection (Struvite) stones.

Technique

For percutaneous nephrostomy see previous section.

Equipment

For dissolving stones, coaxial self-retaining lavage sets are available (Cook; Fig. 2.7), or can be fashioned. The inner pigtail catheter is self-retaining and allows for infusion of irrigant whilst the outer sheath allows for adequate drainage of the fluid to the exterior.

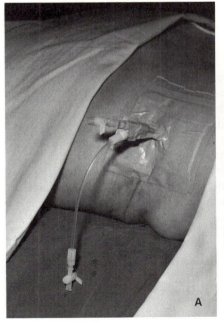
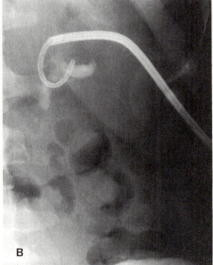

Fig. 2.7 Dissolving stones. (A) Coaxial lavage set. Irrigation through the outer sheath and drainage through the central coaxial pigtail catheter. (B) Cystine stones with lavage set in position.

Irrigation fluids

1. For uric acid and cystine stones:

8.4% sodium bicarbonate	300 ml
Normal saline	700 ml
	1000 ml

2. For cystine stones, 100 ml of 20% acetylcysteine (Mucomyst) is added to each litre.
   The aim is to maintain the urine pH above 7.4. High fluid intake of 5–6 l per day is necessary, and may require intravenous administration.
3. For infection stones (Struvite): 10% solution of hemiacidrin (Renacidin) in water.

   All solutions are run at 100 ml/h using the coaxial lavage system (Fig. 2.7). Check nephrostograms to monitor stone reduction. Mechanical extraction may be used for stone residues.

Ureteric stones

For stones in the upper ureter radiological methods of extraction are an acceptable alternative to lithotripsy and can be performed with a high success rate. The method is particularly useful if nephrostomy is performed because of severe colic or infection.

Equipment

1. A retractable helical stone extractor (Cook Urological, Spencer, Ind.) is used. The 4 wire basket measures 2.2 cm when open and is relatively stiff and expansible (Fig. 2.8). The 0.97 mm (0.038 in) Teflon filiform tip is 20 cm long and a graduated 6F sheath encloses the basket wires during introduction.
2. Amplatz or similar nephrostomy tract dilator set.
3. A 20F or 24F Teflon sheath for insertion into the renal pelvis.
4. A 14F catheter with side arm Tuohy–Borst connector for introducing the extractor coaxially and for injection of fluids.

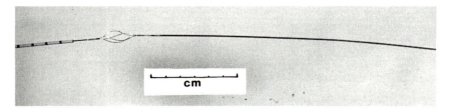

Fig. 28 The 4 wire basket extractor with 20 cm Teflon filiform tip and 6F sheath.

Patient preparation

1. A preliminary percutaneous nephrostomy.
2. Dilatation of the nephrostomy tract to the required size according to the dimensions of the ureteric stone. A Teflon sheath is placed with its tip above the pelviureteric junction.
3. Heavy IV sedation and analgesia with local anaesthesia is necessary for the manipulations. Epidural or general anaesthesia is not usually required.

Technique

1. Using a general purpose curved catheter through the nephrostomy sheath a 0.97 mm (0.038 in) guidewire is manipulated past the ureteric stone.
2. The 6 French extractor sheath is passed over the guidewire to lie beyond the stone.

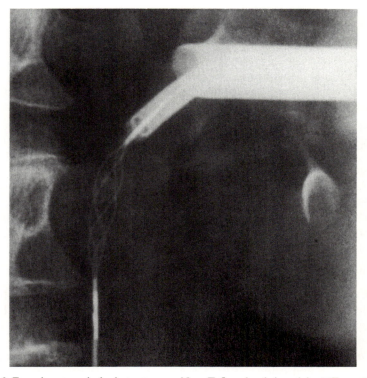

Fig. 2.9 Engaging stone in basket extractor. Note Teflon sheath in pelvis, 14F coaxial catheter used to close basket and to inject fluids. The 6F basket extractor sheath has been retracted.

3. The basket extractor is passed through the sheath with the filiform tip lying in the bladder or near it. The 14F catheter is then passed over the extractor sheath and can be used for injecting contrast.
4. The basket is then exposed to engage the stone which is then locked in position using the tip of the 14F coaxial catheter (Fig. 2.9). The stone is then extracted to the exterior. The extractor sheath is advanced beyond the site of the stone impaction, the extractor is removed and over a guidewire a stenting drainage catheter is introduced and left for several days.

Difficulties and complications

1. Mucosal oedema develops during manipulation of ureteric stones making wall perforation more likely. The long filiform tip overcomes the problem as it always remains in the lumen below the stone.
2. Dropping the stone during removal requires further manipulation but is of no consequence as the nephrostomy sheath prevents the stone escaping into the perirenal tissues.

PLACEMENT OF URETERIC STENTS

Stenting catheters are of two types:
   1. External draining stent. The catheter stenting the ureter passes to the exterior through a nephrostomy track.
   2. Indwelling stent. The catheter is entirely contained within the urinary tract with no external drainage.

Indications

To overcome ureteric obstruction:
   1. Temporary. To provide drainage for obstructions which are reversible, e.g. healing anastomoses or fistulae.
   2. Permanent. Usually to overcome malignant neoplastic ureteric obstruction.

Equipment

   1. External draining stent. It is usual to fashion the stent from a straight polyethylene catheter, 40 cm in length. Multiple side holes are punched so as to lie above and below the ureteric lesion. The tip of the catheter which is usually placed in the bladder should be fashioned into a pigtail.
   2. Indwelling stent. Double-J pigtail multi-holed stents are available of varying length and calibre (VPI, Cook).
   Note: The stent length is specified by measuring the shaft and does not include the pigtail ends.

Patient preparation

1. Percutaneous nephrostomy is performed.
2. Intravenous sedation and analgesia required as the lower urinary tract is particularly sensitive.

Technique

External draining stent

1. The percutaneous nephrostomy catheter is replaced by an end hole polyethylene catheter. If a Cope self-retaining loop nephrostomy tube was used the thread must be divided prior to removal and a straight guide, not a small J, used to straighten the loop.
2. The end hole catheter is manipulated into the ureter with a J guidewire projecting from the tip.
3. The guide and catheter are manipulated through the obstruction, if possible, and passed to the bladder. In very tight obstructions a straight guidewire may be necessary to pass through the narrowed segment. To avoid removing the guidewire for contrast injections, a side arm Tuohy–Borst connection should be attached to the outer end of the catheter and a single side hole made 1 cm proximal to the tip. Sometimes the guide can be passed to the bladder but even the smallest catheter cannot pass the obstruction. In these cases a urethral catheter can be passed and the tip of the ureteric guidewire snared from below and taken to the exterior via the urethra. With an assistant holding the wire taut it is usually possible to force a stenting catheter through the narrowed segment.
4. The end-hole catheter is now replaced by a catheter of similar size with multiple side holes placed so as to lie above and below the obstruction.
5. The catheter is drained externally into a bag.

Indwelling double-J stent

1. Place a temporary external stent with the pigtail in the bladder. This is left for 24 hours or more to be sure that the patient can tolerate the bladder catheter tip. If the external end of the stent is clipped off there is the opportunity to assess the patient's bladder function before introducing the far less easily retrievable internal stent.
2. To measure the length of the internal stent (Fig. 2.10A). A guidewire is passed down the externally draining catheter so that the tip lies at the level of the bladder base. The point of emergence of the guidewire from the external orifice of the catheter is then marked. The guidewire is then withdrawn until the tip lies at a level in the renal pelvis. A second mark is made on the guidewire at the external orifice of the catheter. The distance between the two marks on the guidewire indicates the length of stent required. Remember in ordering that the length of internal

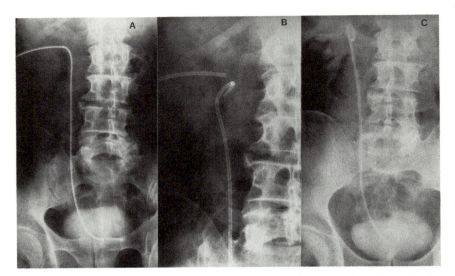

Fig. 2.10 Placement of ureteric stent. (A) Guidewire and catheter tips placed in the bladder prior to measuring the desired length of stent. (B) After removal of guidewire the pusher catheter and the upper end of the stent lie in the pelvis. A nylon suture passes out through the nephrostomy tract to allow final manipulation. (C) Stent in position.

stents does not include the pigtail loops at each end. Also, experience has shown that stent measurement made with the patient prone tends to be too long by about 1 or 2 cm.

3. To insert the internal stent. A stiff guidewire, of Amplatz or Lunder-quist type, is passed through the stent catheter to the bladder and the catheter removed. A nylon suture is looped through two side holes in the upper end of the shaft of the stent to assist minor adjustment. The stent is then passed over the stiff guidewire. When the upper end of the stent reaches the skin surface, the stent is further advanced using a short pusher catheter threaded over the wire. The pusher is provided in some stent sets but can be fashioned simply from a length of PE tubing. The stent is advanced until the upper pigtail end is almost completely in the upper ureter and the lower end of the stent well into the bladder. The guidewire is then removed leaving the tip of the pusher catheter in the renal pelvis and the free ends of the suture out through the nephrostomy tract (Fig. 2.10B).

4. Adjusting the position of the stent. Traction on the suture through the stent allows the upper end to be drawn into the renal pelvis and the pigtail to reform. The suture is then removed by pulling on one end of the loop. Contrast is then injected through the pusher catheter to document the final situation. The pusher is removed and a dressing placed over the nephrostomy incision (Fig. 2.10C).

Difficulties and complications

A wide range of complications have been reported from stents. With a blocked stent it may be possible to withdraw the lower end from the urethra using a cystoscope and to unblock it with a guidewire or replace it with a new stent. It is important that the upper pigtail should be curved in the pelvis. A straight upper end may perforate the kidney substance in time possibly causing a perirenal collection.

RENAL CYST PUNCTURE

Indications

1. To diagnose an indeterminate renal mass when preliminary tests suggest cyst most likely.
2. To treat by ablation cysts causing symptoms, e.g. pain or central cysts interfering with renal function by pressure.

Equipment

For localization

1. For IVP localization. Metal skin marker. Ureteric compression belt.
2. For ultrasound localization. Mobile real time scanner.
3. Needle 20 gauge and 10 cm long. Connecting tube. Syringe (20 ml).
4. Contrast medium. Low viscosity and easily miscible, e.g. Retroconray (M&B).

Patient preparation

Local anaesthesia.

Technique

1. Patient prone over a firm bolster. Ureteric compression band in situ comfortably tight if using IVP for localization.
2. Localize cyst, using IVP and fluoroscopy or ultrasound. Mark skin vertically over cyst. If using X-rays, centre on the metal skin marker when filming to avoid parallax error.
3. Inject local anaesthesia after skin sterilization. Infiltrate to renal capsule.
4. Pass puncture needle attached to syringe by connecting tube to renal capsule during suspended respiration. When the capsule is entered the needle swings with respiration.
5. Check direction with fluoroscopy or ultrasound.
6. Advance needle whilst applying suction. Straw-coloured fluid is obtained when a simple cyst is entered.
7. Inject contrast under fluoroscopy. Make films in various projections.

Difficulties and complications

1. Confirming a diagnosis of benign cyst. Straw-coloured aspirate makes the diagnosis for practical purposes and analysis of fluid is not necessary. Bloody aspirate is suspicious of tumour. Important to check with films that the contrast-filled cyst accounts for the entire space lesion. Sometimes a simple cyst may be closely adjacent to a tumour.
2. Limited aspirate. Sometimes the aspiration of straw-coloured fluid ceases after a small amount is removed. Do not alter the needle position but inject some contrast medium, which will almost always outline the cyst cavity.

Treating a simple renal cyst

Numerous methods have been advocated but injection of absolute alcohol seems the best. The majority of cysts do not require treatment.

Principle

After aspirating the cyst completely introduce a volume of alcohol equal to about 25% of the cyst volume. After 20 minutes aspirate the alcohol from the cyst.

Equipment

1. 10 cm needle to take 0.89 mm (0.035 in) guidewire.
2. 5F polyethylene end hole catheter 15 cm long. Using boiling water shape a tight pigtail tip.
3. Ampoules of 100% dehydrated alcohol (BP).
4. 1 ampoule of oily contrast medium (Pantopaque or Myodil).

Technique

1. As for cyst puncture introduce needle into cyst.
2. Using a 0.89 mm (0.035 in) guide replace needle with 5F pigtail catheter. Place catheter well into the cyst. Outline cyst with contrast (Fig. 2.11A). Assess approximate volume of cyst from radiographs.
3. Aspirate cyst completely if possible. The pigtail will prevent withdrawal of catheter tip from cyst (Fig. 2.11B). Inject a volume of alcohol equal to 25% of estimated volume.
4. Leave for 20 minutes, then aspirate. Inject 1–2 ml of Pantopaque or Myodil as future marker of cyst size. Remove catheter.

Difficulties and complications

1. Alcohol absorption. This is not a problem.

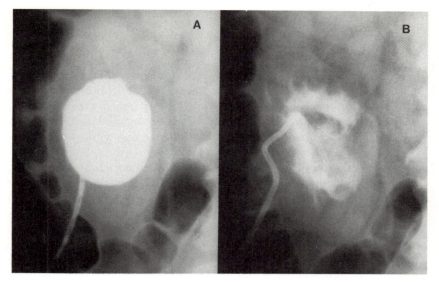

Fig. 2.11 Alcohol treatment of renal cyst. (A) Cyst outlined with contrast to assess volume. (B) After aspiration prior to alcohol injection. Note pigtail catheter well contained within the collapsed cyst.

2. Cyst reforms. This is a common occurrence. A further injection should be performed.

CYSTOGRAPHY

The bladder may be outlined by urethral catheter, the usual route, or on occasions by suprapubic puncture. Cystography may also be performed as part of intravenous pyelography.

Indications

1. To demonstrate bladder pathology, e.g. diverticula, tumours, etc.
2. Preliminary to micturating studies of vesicoureteric reflux or urethral pathology.
3. To detect bladder injury following trauma.
4. To study stress incontinence.

Equipment

Nothing special.

Patient preparation

Urethral anaesthesia with 1% xylocaine jelly if urethral catheterization is used. The bladder should be moderately distended prior to suprapubic puncture.

Technique

1. Urethral catheterization is the usual means of filling the bladder with contrast medium. The procedure should be performed with meticulous asepsis. After anaesthetizing the urethra a moderate-sized pliable side hole catheter should be introduced to the bladder using a 'no touch' technique employing forceps.
2. For suprapubic puncture the moderately distended bladder should be identified by palpation or preferably by ultrasound. Puncture is made just above the pubis in the midline after infiltrating local anaesthetic. A catheter-sheathed needle combination, gauge 19, is directed 10° cranially to enter the bladder and the needle is then moved. Moderate bladder distension is important as it elevates the anterior peritoneal reflection so that the puncture is made extra peritoneally. In infants, bladder distension may be achieved by hydration or diuretic.
3. Remember that with the patient supine during pyelography only the posterior half of the bladder is outlined by the denser than urine contrast medium. Rolling the patient is necessary to ensure that the entire bladder, including the urachal extension is evenly opacified.
4. AP and both oblique views are necessary to demonstrate filling defects and abnormalities of contour.
5. To demonstrate the prostatic impression an AP view with cranial angulation (12°) of the X-ray beam, centred on the symphysis pubis is useful.
6. To demonstrate cystocele a very slightly obliqued lateral view of the pelvis is made erect with and without the patient straining. A similar view is used to demonstrate the female urethra during micturition.
7. Demonstration of vesico-ureteric reflux in adults is best using a fluoroscope with the patient standing erect or sitting on a commode chair. It is essential to make films which include the entire urinary tract, particularly the pelvicalyceal systems. In young infants the study is made supine and the bladder is filled until the baby spontaneously micturates around the catheter when filming of the upper tracts is made to detect reflux.

Difficulties and complications

1. Failure to void on request. This is a common problem particularly if the bladder is underfilled.
2. Use of too dense a medium may obscure filling defects.
3. Developmental abnormalities or strictures may preclude filling of the bladder per urethra.
4. Suprapubic bladder puncture frequently causes transient micro haematuria but with ultrasound control significant complications should not

occur. Transperitoneal puncture has resulted in bowel perforation and peritonitis.

URETHROGRAPHY AND PASSAGE OF STRICTURES

The urethra may be demonstrated by retrograde injection of contrast or in antegrade fashion during micturition, having opacified the bladder urine.

Indications

1. To demonstrate obstructive lesions. Retrograde injection is used to demonstrate strictures, ruptures, filling defects and prostatic abnormalities. Antegrade technique is valuable in children to demonstrate valves and in adults may show obstruction.
2. Following severe pelvic trauma to assess the integrity of the urethra prior to passage of a catheter.

Equipment

1. Retrograde. A device for pressure injecting the urethra, without leakage, is required. The urethral cage and cannula, first described by Brodny in 1941, in our experience is still the most effective in males (Fig. 2.12). The Knuttson clamp is also popular but leakage frequently occurs. A small Foley balloon catheter may be used and is best for females.
2. A viscous water soluble contrast medium such as Endografin (Schering) is preferred.

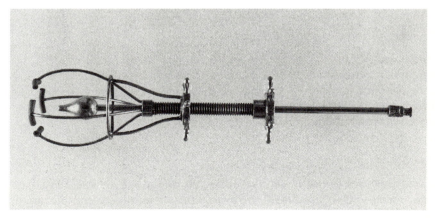

Fig. 2.12 Brodny urethrography equipment. The outer cage compresses the base of the glans. The coaxial metal cannula is inserted in the urethra and locked in position.

Patient preparation

The urethra is filled with xylocaine 1% jelly which is also smeared on the glans prior to application of the clamp.

Technique

1. AP and oblique views are made demonstrating the entire length of the urethra. Films are made during filling to obtain maximal distention.
2. Dilute water soluble contrast medium is introduced to outline the bladder prior to the antegrade study. With the male patient erect and slightly oblique, spot films are made during micturition, using a fluoroscope.
3. Following pelvic trauma and before attempts at bladder catheterization contrast is injected and a film is exposed to assess urethral rupture. Further views are made according to the findings.
4. Occasionally bladder filling with contrast, prior to antegrade urethrography is performed by suprapubic puncture.

Difficulties and complications

1. Occasionally minor congenital abnormalities prevent adequate attachment of the injection device. Use of the small Foley balloon type catheter will usually overcome the problem.
2. Extravasation of contrast medium using water soluble contrast may occur with venous filling and is of no consequence. Oily media were at one time used and oil embolism sometimes occurred.
3. Urethral spasm. Posterior urethral spasm may prevent contrast entering the bladder. Adequate anaesthesia of the urethra usually overcomes the problem, but rarely parenteral sedation and analgesis may be required.

Passage of tight urethral strictures

Radiological techniques provide an atraumatic means of passage of tight urethral strictures which defy blind instrumentation. Passage of the stricture is required prior to internal urethrotomy or balloon dilatation. The passage can be performed in retrograde fashion from below or from above after performing suprapubic puncture.

Retrograde passage of stricture

A moderate-sized pliable end hole catheter, about 14F in size, with a side arm Tuohy–Borst attachment is selected. After anaesthetizing the urethra with xylocaine jelly 1% the catheter, of sufficient size to largely fill the urethra, is introduced to the level of stricture. Under fluoroscopic control and injecting contrast medium through the side arm of the connector the narrow channel through the stricture is probed using a straight guidewire. After successfully passing the guidewire to the posterior urethra a smaller tapered dilating catheter is substituted for the larger catheter and passed upwards to the bladder.

Antegrade passage of urethral stricture

After introducing a catheter into the bladder under local anaesthesia suprapubically, the track is dilated to allow introduction of either a steer-able Meditec type catheter or a sharply curved 10 French catheter. Taking care not to irritate the sensitive trigone the catheter tip is directed to the urethral orifice at the bladder neck. Once the urethra is entered a straight guidewire is passed down through the stricture, which is outlined by contrast introduced through a sidearm on the catheter system. The guide-wire is advanced to the exterior so that both ends of the guidewire can be controlled (Fig. 2.13). This arrangement allows dilating catheters to be introduced from above to dilate the urethral stricture. Balloon dilatation can also be performed or the guidewire can be left in position to guide the urologist whilst performing internal urethrotomy.

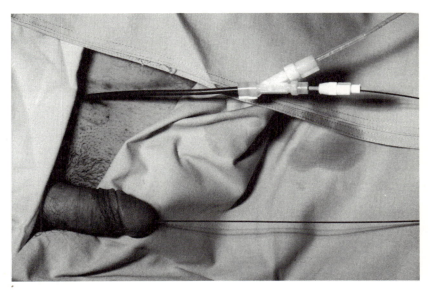

Fig. 2.13 Guidewire entering the bladder suprapubically through an 8.3F catheter and sheath set and emerging from the external penile meatus.

REFERENCES

Ansell G 1976 Complications in diagnostic radiology. London Blackwell Scientific Publishers
Lasser E C, Berry C C, Talner L B et al 1987 Pretreatment with corticosteroids to alleviate reactions to intravenous contrast material. New England Journal of Medicine 317: 845–849
Whitaker R H 1979 The Whitaker test. Urologic Clinics of North America 6: 529–532

FURTHER READING

Bean W J 1981 Renal cysts: treatment with alcohol. Radiology 138: 329–331
Brodny M L 1941 A new instrument for urethrography in the male. Journal of Urology
46: 350–354
Cope C 1980 Improved anchoring of nephrostomy catheters: loop technique. American Journal
of Roentgenology 135: 402–403
Cope C, Zeit R 1982 Pseudoaneurysms after nephrostomy. American Journal of Roentgenology
139: 255–261
Dretler S, Pfister R, Newhouse J 1979 Renal stone dissolution via percutaneous nephrostomy.
New England Journal of Medicine 300: 341–343
Gerber W L, Narayana A S 1982 Failure of the double-curved ureteral stent. Journal of
Urology 127: 317–319
Hare W S C, McOmish D 1981 Skinny needle pyelography: an advance in uroradiology.
Medical Journal of Australia 12: 123–125
Hare W S C, McOmish D 1982 Nephrostomy lavage set for dissolving renal stones. Radiology
144: 932
Hare W S C, McOmish D, Nunn I N 1981 Percutaneous transvesical antegrade passage of
urethral strictures. Urologic Radiology 3: 107–112
McOmish D, Hare W S C 1982 Antegrade urography: the use of oily contrast material.
Radiology 144: 933–934
Marberger M, Stackl W, Hruby W 1982 Percutaneous litholapaxy of renal calculi with
ultrasound. European Urology 8: 236–242
Pass R F, Waldo F B 1979 Anaerobic bacteremia following suprapubic bladder aspiration.
Journal of Pediatrics 94: 748
Wickham J, Kellett M, Miller R 1983 Elective percutaneous nephrolithotomy in 50 patients:
an analysis of the technique, results and complications. Urology 129: 904–906.

3

Gastrointestinal and biliary tracts

BARIUM SULPHATE PREPARATIONS

The precise recipes for commercially available preparations are trade secrets. Most are suspensions of barium sulphate with a fine particle size of less than 1.0 μm. These fine particles are produced by precipitation from solution rather than by grinding naturally occurring barite ores — the older method which resulted in coarser particles. The two most important factors determining the results produced by barium are the suspension stability and the coating ability on mucosal surfaces. Barium sulphate is commonly maintained in suspension by incorporating a naturally occurring gum, a pectin or cellulose derivative. The effect is produced by the long chain molecules in these suspending agents forming weak bonds with each other and with the surface of the barium particles. Small particle size also helps the suspending ability. Maintaining barium sulphate particles in suspension at low density, such as the 15% w/v ratio often used for single contrast barium enemas, is considerably more difficult than at the higher densities used for upper bowel studies. The coating ability of barium sulphate is dependent on many factors but one of the most important is the viscosity. At any given density of barium, the thicker the mucosal coating the more opaque it is, and the thickness of the coating at any point depends upon the viscosity. However, high viscosity barium suspensions can be shown to obscure surface detail such as the areae gastricae. The optimal compromise has been found to be a high density of low viscosity. This produces a less easily maintained film but one capable of showing surface detail.

Many barium preparations are available, but each should be selected for the role it is required to play.

BARIUM MEAL

Many methods for performing this study have been described and the one outlined here is the author's preference. All barium meals should use a double contrast technique with gas. Single contrast studies are only acceptable in patients so debilitated that only a limited study is possible. The

35

essence of a good barium meal is that all areas should be examined, first barium filled and then gas filled.

Preparation

1. The patient should fast from solids for at least 4 hours and preferably 12 hours before the examination. Clear fluids may be taken up to 2 hours before.
2. The optimum barium preparation has a high density and low viscosity, such as a EZHD, where 70 ml of water are added to 340 g of powder to produce a 240% w/v suspension.
3. Some commercially available barium preparations require a small amount of simethicone bubble breaker. This is to disperse gas bubbles from the barium since these may otherwise be confused with polyps in the stomach.
4. To gain a double contrast effect gas must be introduced into the stomach. Most commercial preparations combine citric acid with sodium bicarbonate, to produce carbon dioxide. The ideal amount of gas is 250 ml since larger amounts may so distend the stomach that the mucosal folds are effaced.

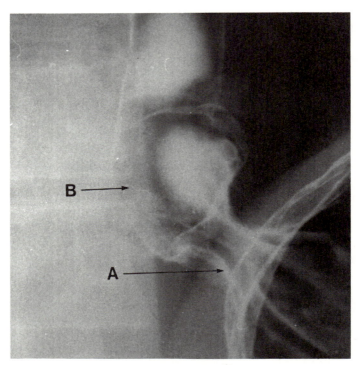

Fig. 3.1 Double contrast oesophagogram demonstrating gastric mucosal folds (A) passing through the diaphragm into a hiatus hernia (B).

5. In order to overcome spasm, particularly in the duodenal cap, a smooth muscle relaxant such as 20 mg IV buscopan (hyoscine) is given routinely. If there is a history of heart disease, prostatic retention or glaucoma, buscopan should not be used. An alternative is glucagon 0.2 mg. If given intravenously the effect is almost instantaneous and lasts for 5–10 minutes. Glucagon has virtually no side effects at this dosage, however with larger doses one should consider the possibility of provoking reactive hypoglycaemia in patients with insulinoma, or hypertension in cases of phaeochromocytoma. Because it wears off quickly it has virtually no effect on small bowel transit time.

Technique

The patient is given the gas producing mixture first, to allow time for CO_2 to form. The smooth muscle relaxant is given next and then approximately 100 ml of barium suspension. The patient is placed on the fluoroscopic table and rolled twice through 360° to coat the gastric walls. With the patient prone and the left side raised, two full length films of the oesophagus are taken. This should be relaxed and air filled, giving a double contrast oesophagogram (Fig. 3.1). With the patient now lying prone over

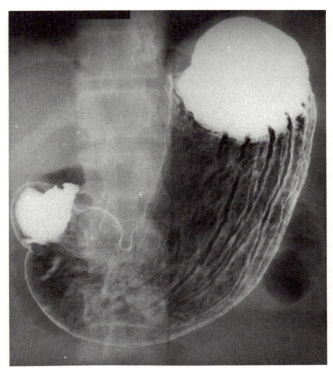

Fig. 3.2 Normal supine view of the stomach at barium meal.

a pillow, the increased intra-abdominal pressure so produced will make a hiatus hernia apparent if it is present. Three full views of the stomach are now taken; prone with left side raised, supine with the right side raised and flat supine (Fig. 3.2). Four views of the duodenal cap are taken, one with the cap barium filled prone, two with the cap air filled (with the patient supine and the right side raised) and finally one view of the gas filled cap with the patient erect. With the patient erect a final full view of the stomach, with the patient turned a little to the left, is taken to view the gas filled fundus.

If the patient is obese or if overlying bowel loops prevent good visualization of particular areas, especially of the duodenal cap, spot films should be taken with a compression device.

OESOPHAGEAL STUDIES

Indications

If patients complain of dysphagia localized to the upper or lower oesophagus, special views must be taken. It is essential in any oesophageal study that the whole length be examined, since lower obstruction may be referred to the neck symptomatically.

Technique

To evaluate motility problems such as scleroderma or 'corkscrew oesophagus', no smooth muscle relaxant is used. The patient is examined prone or supine to neutralize the effect of gravity and a fluoroscopic evaluation of peristalsis is made. In patients with high dysphagia, rapid sequence filming, such as two frames per second, is desirable with two runs AP and two laterally to determine the constancy or otherwise of any abnormality. In cases of low dysphagia an examination of the fundus of the stomach must be included, since lower oesophageal carcinomas may originate there. In all cases of dysphagia it is very useful to have the patient swallow barium soaked bread or marshmallow in order to reproduce symptoms. In all these examinations the barium preparation is as for a double contrast meal.

Gastro-oesophageal reflux

This is best demonstrated supine with barium in the gastric fundus. As the patient rolls slowly to the right the bolus of barium will cross the oesophago-gastric junction and reflux may be reproduced.

Oesophageal rupture or fistula

If there is a likelihood of communication between the oesophagus and mediastinal tissues, a water soluble contrast medium such as Gastrografin (sodium meglumine diatrizoate) with a single contrast technique is used. Gastrografin is rapidly absorbed from the tissues, whereas barium sets up a chemical inflammation. If a communication with the bronchial tree is suspected, bronchographic contrast medium such as Dionosil is used for a single contrast swallow. While barium in the bronchial tree is not disastrous and may be coughed up without incident, Gastrografin by virtue of its hygroscopic effect, may cause severe pulmonary oedema in adults, and death in infants, if allowed into the bronchial tree.

Hypotonic duodenography

This technique is now largely outdated with the widespread use of endoscopic and CT evaluation of the pancreas. It may, however, be used in evaluation of known disease of the second part of duodenum or in the superior mesenteric artery syndrome. The method is as for a double contrast barium meal except that the smooth muscle relaxant is given when the second part of the duodenum is full of barium. The patient is then placed supine with the right side raised. This will drain barium from the second part of duodenum and fill it with gas. A double contrast effect is thus produced, and spot films in various degrees of obliquity are taken (Fig. 3.3).

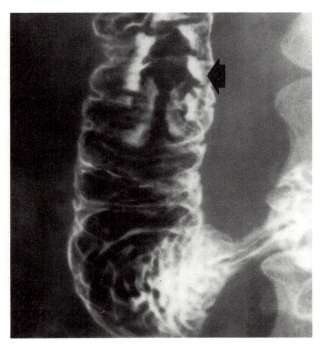

Fig. 3.3 Hypotonic duodenogram showing an abnormally large ampulla of Vater (arrow) containing a hamartoma.

SMALL BOWEL STUDIES

Indications

Barium studies of the small bowel may be performed to diagnose the presence and nature of malabsorption states, the extent of inflammatory or malignant disease and the level of obstructions. The examination can be performed either as part of an oral follow through study or as a small bowel enema if a double contrast effect is required.

Patient preparation

The patient should not eat on the morning of the examination. Oral clear fluids may be taken up to 2 hours prior to the study. It is useful to give the patient a mild aperient the night before the examination as a clean colon facilitates barium transit of the small bowel.

The barium follow-through

The conventional double contrast barium meal, if performed beforehand should use no smooth muscle relaxant, although glucagon has little effect on small bowel transit time. In addition to the 100 ml of high density barium used for the meal, a further 150 ml of more dilute barium is given. This can be made by adding 120 ml of water to a standard pack of barium (about 300 g) instead of the usual 70 ml. It is most important that the large volume (250 ml) of barium is given since smaller amounts, by not giving a continuous contrast column to fill the small bowel, may result in a misleading appearance of flocculation and an incorrect diagnosis of malabsorption state. Ideally, the patient should have multiple spot films of individual small bowel loops with compression and in particular, views of the terminal ileum. Full length abdomen films should be taken every 30 minutes until the colon begins to be opacified. Obviously, if a partial or complete small bowel obstruction is present, the films will have to be at considerably longer intervals.

Pitfalls

1. All full-length abdomen films in small bowel studies should include the symphysis pubis. The reason for this is to avoid missing a fistula between the small bowel and sigmoid with premature rectal opacification. This is a not infrequent occurrence in patients with Crohn's disease.
2. Underfilling of the small bowel is a common cause for the radiological misdiagnosis of malabsorption state.

Small bowel enema

A naso-duodenal tube of about 10 French, such as a Bilbao–Dotter type, is passed through the nose down to the stomach. This tube has a central removable stiffening wire which terminates in a broad 'J' curve. With the patient lying on the right side the tip of the 'J' is directed to the pyloric canal and the tube fed off this into the duodenum. The optimal position for the tip is at the duodenal–jejunal flexure and this position can be checked fluoroscopically. 100 ml of thick barium (240% w/v as for a double contrast barium meal) are now instilled down the tube. This is followed slowly by 2 l of luke warm gelatin solution, made by mixing 10 g of powdered gelatin in hot water. In this way a double contrast effect is produced and the gelatin does not wash the barium off the small bowel mucosa. This volume of fluid is usually sufficient to chase the barium down to the caecum. Spot films of each loop of small bowel and a final overcouch, full abdomen film are obtained.

Small bowel obstruction

In patients with partial bowel obstruction many surgeons prefer the use of water soluble contrast such as gastrografin which has a lubricating effect in overcoming partial obstruction.

BARIUM ENEMA

Indications

While the single contrast or 'full column' barium enema was popular until recent years, its insensitivity in detection of small colonic lesions has meant that it now is only suitable as a means of the retrograde identification of the site of colon obstruction or as a cautious exploration of the length of colonic involvement in a patient with fulminating ulcerative colitis. For most other purposes a double contrast technique should be used.

Contraindications

1. Toxic megacolon is usually a contraindication to barium enema. However, after close consultation with the managing physicians, a cautious single contrast study may be indicated to show the proximal extent of ulceration in a patient with active colitis. The risk of perforating the bowel is high.
2. Full thickness bowel wall biopsy in the preceding 24 hours is an absolute contraindication.
3. Recent pelvic irradiation is associated with radiation colitis and may lead to bowel perforation.
4. A bowel that is incompletely cleansed makes the barium enema

practically useless apart from the detection of the grossest lesions. Worse than this, substantial lesions may be overlooked or attributed to faecal contamination, and the study called normal. Such patients with an inadequately cleansed bowel must be rebooked after thorough cleansing. This is the responsibility of the radiologist and not of the referring clinician.

Preparation

1. The patient should fast from solid food for 24 hours prior to the examination. Clear fluids or jelly may be taken during this period.
2. The patient should be given an aperient the night before the examination. A suitable regimen is 40 g magnesium citrate powder mixed with water, four 5 mg tablets of bisacodyl all taken the evening before the study and then one 10 mg bisacodyl suppository the following morning. This should ideally be followed by a 2 l clear water enema on arrival in the radiology clinic.

Barium sulphate suspensions for double contrast enemas

The radiologist must experiment with the barium preparation which best suits his purpose. The ideal barium should have high density, a good flow rate and be resistant to drying on the colonic mucosa. The usual density will be 60% w/v.

Technique

The following is a modification of the 'seven pump method' described by Miller and Maglinte. With the patient in a left lateral position the enema tube is inserted in the rectum. An inflatable cuff should be used if the patient is likely to be rectally incontinent. The patient is turned prone and the barium is run in from a bag elevated one metre above the table top. As soon as the barium has reached the transverse colon the rectal tube is clamped and air is inflated into the colon through the enema tube, in a sequence of seven pumps on a sphygmomanometer bulb, in each of seven positions:
1. Lateral, left side down.
2. Prone oblique, right side elevated.
3. Prone.
4. Prone oblique, left side elevated.
5. Lateral, right side down.
6. Supine oblique, left side elevated.
7. Supine.
The patient is now turned prone and the table head elevated 45°, to drain

the rectum and sigmoid and to bring more barium into the caecum. Following drainage, the table is returned to horizontal and seven more pumps of air are instilled with the patient prone. This entire procedure will usually require 63 to 70 pumps on a sphygmomanometer bulb. The following sequence of films are taken:
1. Prone 30 × 25 cm film of the recto sigmoid with the X-ray tube directed 15° toward the feet.
2. Prone oblique, left side raised 30 × 25 cm film of the recto sigmoid with X-ray tube directed 15° toward the feet.
3. Lateral 30 × 25 cm film of the rectum with the right side up.
4. Erect oblique 30 × 25 cm film of the splenic and hepatic flexures (each separately).
5. Erect AP 36 × 36 cm film of the transverse colon.
6. Supine AP 36 × 54 cm film of the whole abdomen.
7. Supine oblique, with first the right and then the left side raised, views of the caecum. These are taken on a 30 × 25 cm film split vertically in two.
8 and 9.
   Right and left lateral decubitus 36 × 54 cm films of the whole abdomen using a horizontal beam.

Complications

1. Inability to fill the terminal ileum in patients suspected of Crohn's disease. A simple manoeuvre is to have the patient evacuate the bowel on the toilet at the end of the procedure. Colonic peristalsis very often will drive barium back into the ileum.
2. Perforation of the bowel is a surgical emergency, as barium sets up an intense chemical inflammation in the peritoneum. This rare complication can be avoided by ensuring that the rectal balloon is not overinflated, that there has been no recent full thickness colon biopsy, and that the patient does not have toxic megacolon.
3. Post procedural constipation is an occasional problem and may be avoided by advising the patient to take liberal oral fluids and perhaps a mild aperient.

THERAPEUTIC BARIUM ENEMA

Indications

In infants an intussusception may be reduced by the cautious use of a barium single contrast enema. The intussusception should not have been present for more than 24 hours, for after that time the bowel may be severely ischaemic and may perforate.

Preparation

1. No patient preparation is necessary.
2. The barium preparation used may be of low density 15% w/v in order to flow freely.

Technique

A fine rubber catheter, without a balloon, is inserted into the rectum and taped to the child's buttocks. The barium container is elevated 90 cm from the table top and barium run through the tubing into the rectum for 3 minutes. The retrograde progress of the barium and the intussusception is monitored fluoroscopically. If the intussusception does not move after 3 minutes the barium flow is turned off. Only 3 such 3 minute-long trials of barium should be attempted if the intussusception is not moving and the procedure should then be abandoned. If the intussusception is moving retrogradely, the barium pressure may be continued until reduction is complete.

COLOSTOMY STUDIES WITH BARIUM

Indications

There are two principal areas of study in patients with a colostomy. Prior to closure of a colostomy the distal limb may need to be evaluated for lumen calibre or for the integrity of an anastomosis. Alternatively a retrograde study may be required to study the bowel proximal to a colostomy.

Preparation

Little or no patient preparation is needed since the proximal limb of a colostomy often contains fluid only, and the distal limb is empty.

Technique

Retrograde enema of the distal limb

1. If no anastomotic leak is considered likely, a simple retrograde single contrast barium enema from the rectum to the colostomy is sufficient.
2. If an anastomotic leak is likely, the retrograde enema from the rectum should be performed using water soluble contrast such as 30% Urografin (sodium meglumine diatrizoate).

Retrograde enema of the proximal limb

Barium can be introduced through a 14F Foley catheter while the patient

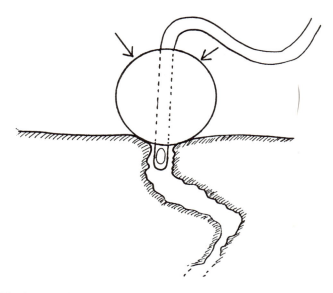

Fig. 3.4 The balloon of a Foley catheter may be held by the patient against the opening of a colostomy to provide a seal during instillation of barium.

holds the balloon tight against the colostomy opening (Fig. 3.4). This will prevent spillage. Air may be introduced through the same route to obtain a double contrast study.

ORAL CHOLECYSTOGRAPHY AND CHOLANGIOGRAPHY

Indications

Oral cholecystography is nowadays regarded as being competitive with ultrasound for gallstone diagnosis. The oral study remains cost effective and if performed carefully has a similar accuracy to ultrasound.

Contraindications

It is usually pointless attempting the study in a jaundiced patient, particularly one with obstructive jaundice.

Preparation

1. A mild aperient such as 1–2 tablets of bisacodyl, should be taken the night before the examination.
2. The night before the examination a fat-free light meal may be taken but no food on the morning of the study. Beverages such as tea should be milk free to avoid stimulating the gallbladder to empty.

Contrast media

A suitable regimen is 3 g sodium ipodate (Biloptin, Schering) the night before the examination and 3 g calcium ipodate (Solu-Biloptin, Schering) the following morning. This has several advantages over other regimens. Firstly, it amounts to a double dose of contrast and a repeat visit is not necessary. Secondly, the Solu-Biloptin, being rapidly excreted in the bile, outlines the common hepatic and common bile ducts, while Biloptin shows the gallbladder.

Radiography

1. All films should be exposed at a low kilo-voltage (55–65 kV). The exposure time should be kept as short as possible, if necessary by shortening the focus film distance.
2. Films may be taken either with an overcouch tube or as fluoroscopic spot films.
3. Whenever possible compression should be used to reduce the thickness of soft tissue. This is particularly important in obese patients.
4. All films should be tightly coned.

Films

The following is the usual sequence of films.
  1. *Plain film*
     The film is usually taken at the time the patient makes their appointment, i.e. before contrast is taken. While this is a traditional part of the oral cholecystogram several series have shown that it very rarely makes a difference to the final diagnosis since most calculi are only lightly calcified and are detectable when the gallbladder is full of contrast. This film may therefore be safely dropped from the series.
  2. *Post contrast films*
   (a) *Prone*: This is the most commonly performed film in that it brings the gallbladder closest to the film. The film may be either flat prone or prone oblique with the right side raised a little. This latter film is particularly useful in thin patients in whom the gallbladder lies medially and must therefore be thrown clear of the spine by this manoeuvre.
   (b) *Supine oblique*: This film is taken with the left side slightly raised since the contrast, being heavier than bile, tends to layer out. The fundus is shown best in the prone view, and the neck and body in the supine. If the gallbladder is low lying, the patient may be tipped slightly head down (Trendelenburg) to separate the gallbladder and colon.
   (c) *Erect*: The advantage of this film, taken with a horizontal beam, is

that it is possible to visualize calculi either fallen to the fundus of the gallbladder or floating in a layer in the bile.

3. Additional views

(d) *Lateral decubitus*: The patient lies on the right side on an elevated padding. A horizontal beam is used, centred to the tip of the twelfth rib.

(e) *Supine angled view*: Here the X-ray tube is angled 20° toward the head with the patient supine, or 20° to the feet prone. This will tend to project the gallbladder above the hepatic flexure.

(f) *After Fatty Meal (AFM)*: This film is taken provided there are no calculi detected in the gallbladder. A bout of biliary pain may otherwise ensue. The patient eats a small bar of milk chocolate and after 20 minutes a single film is taken in the optimal position chosen from among the pre AFM films.

Complications

Failure of the gallbladder to opacify adequately

1. Tomography should be performed in this situation and may give a conclusive diagnosis in what appears a hopeless situation. Tomography will also more clearly define the bile duct.
2. If tomography is unsuccessful, we routinely refer the patient to ultrasound. We have not found repeat studies useful and without regimen the patient has already had the equivalent of a double dose of contrast.
3. Contrast reactions of a serious nature are very rare. Nausea, vomiting and diarrhoea are quite common, however, and may contribute to non-absorption of the contrast.

INTRAVENOUS CHOLANGIOGRAPHY

Indications

This procedure is particularly to demonstrate the biliary tree in the post cholecystectomy patient. With the wide use of ERCP it is only infrequently performed.

Contraindications

1. Allergy to intravenous contrast media.
2. Significant jaundice unless it is falling.
3. Recent oral cholecystogram. There is some evidence to suggest a greater incidence of severe reactions to IVC in patients who have had an oral study in the preceding 24 hours but not after this. The two studies should therefore not be performed on the same day.

Preparation

1. The patient should take fluids only on the morning of the study.
2. A mild aperient such as 1–2 tablets of bisacodyl should be given the night before the study.
3. Plentiful oral fluids should be taken to reduce the risk of renal damage by contrast. This is particularly important in patients with renal failure.

Contrast medium

1. The most common medium is 20 ml Biligrafin forte (Iodipamide-Schering) given by slow intravenous injection. The slowness of the injection (over 5 minutes) is important because a rapid injection will produce nausea and vomiting in most patients.
2. Biligrafin is also available as a 200 ml solution for drip infusion.
3. A recent and promising contrast medium is Biliscopin. This is reputed to have significantly fewer side effects than Biligrafin. It is given as a 100 ml drip infusion.

Technique

Contrast is most dense 30–45 minutes after injection and is fading by 60 minutes. Tomographic slices are therefore taken at 30 minutes with the patient supine and the left side raised a little. It is usual to find the duct at 11–13 cm from the back. Several 1 cm thick slices will be required since the entire duct will not be seen on any one.

OPERATIVE CHOLANGIOGRAPHY

Indications

Operative cholangiography is performed during cholecystectomy to exclude the presence of bile duct calculi. It may be performed before or after manual exploration of the duct.

Equipment

1. The head of the X-ray machine requires a sterile cover.
2. A tunnel beneath the operating table is required to allow film cassettes to be changed.
3. Suitable contrast medium is 30% Urografin (sodium meglumine diatrizoate). The concentration must be low in order that small calculi are not obscured.

Technique

Pre-exploration

1. The surgeon cannulates the cystic duct with fine plastic tubing such as a ureteric catheter.
2. A 20 ml syringe of contrast is attached to the catheter end and bile is aspirated to ensure an air bubble free system.
3. The table is tilted 15° to the right and the radiographer centres the X-ray table to the cystic duct junction to the common bile duct. This point is indicated by the surgeon.
4. All metal instruments are removed from the area of the exposure.
5. It is usual to take 3 films, one each after the surgeon has slowly injected 3 ml, 8 ml and 12 ml of contrast.
6. Each film is exposed in suspended respiration as controlled by the anaesthetist.

Post-exploration

The same procedure as the above is carried out when the T-tube has been sewn in the place of the cystic duct catheter.

Complications

1. Air bubbles can largely be avoided if the surgeon injects the contrast with the syringe vertical and the plunger uppermost.

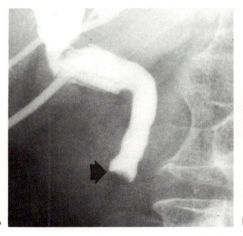
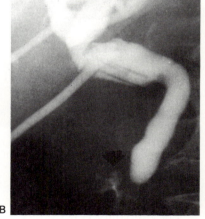

A   B

Fig. 3.5 The pseudocalculus demonstrated during T-tube cholangiography. In (A) the initial film shows a contracted sphincter of Oddi (arrow) giving a false impression of a calculus in the distal common bile duct. In (B) a few moments later a wave of contraction has passed and contrast is now seen in the duodenum (arrow).

2. Failure of contrast to enter the duodenum. This complication is commonly due to the oedema of the sphincter of Oddi as a result of the surgeon's exploration. If the distal bile duct tapers to a point, such an appearance can be accepted as normal.
3. Pseudocalculus is the term applied to a concave inferior end of the common bile duct sometimes caused by contraction of the sphincter of Oddi. On a single film this may exactly simulate a calculus, but on a serial film the wave of contraction will be seen to pass (Fig. 3.5).

T-TUBE CHOLANGIOGRAPHY

Indications

This examination is for the detection of any calculi left in the biliary tree after cholecystectomy.

Contrast medium

Urografin 30% (sodium meglumine diatrizoate) is suitable. A low concentration is used so that small calculi are not obscured by the contrast (Fig. 3.6).

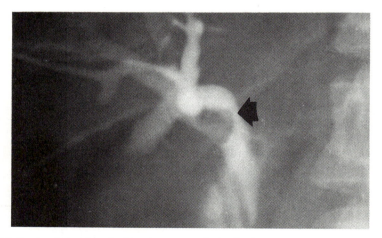

Fig. 3.6 T-tube cholangiogram demonstrates a calculus in the common hepatic duct (arrow).

Technique

1. The procedure is performed under fluoroscopic control and the patient lies supine on the table.
2. The external part of the T-tube is clamped approximately 30 cm (1 ft) from the skin.

3. The portion of tube between the skin and the clamp is sterilized and laid on a sterile towel.
4. A syringe with 20 ml of contrast and a 21 gauge needle attached is carefully cleared of air bubbles. The needle is inserted through the wall of the rubber tube. Bile is gently drawn back into the syringe to ensure an air bubble free system.
5. Several coned views of the bile ducts including the distal end are taken in different degrees of obliquity while contrast is being gently injected.
6. It is most important that the junction of the common bile duct with the duodenum is clearly identified and projected free from other bowel loops.
7. Finally, a supine 30 × 24 cm film including the intrahepatic ducts is taken. All films are carefully scrutinized before the patient gets off the table. If the presence of calculi is not clear, more films must be taken to resolve the issue.

Complications

Air bubbles in the biliary tree are a difficult diagnostic problem. Obviously every effort should be made to keep them out of the tubing. If they are present, however, a useful manoeuvre is to tilt the table into the erect position. Lucencies due to air bubbles will usually float upwards. Calculi tend to sink to a lower level.

ENDOSCOPIC RETROGRADE CHOLANGIO-PANCREATOGRAPHY (ERCP)

Indications

ERCP is becoming an increasingly valuable technique for evaluation of the ampulla of Vater, the pancreatic duct and biliary tree. In the pancreatic system its indications are the identification of duct irregularities seen in neoplasm or chronic inflammation. Pseudocysts of the pancreas will fill from the ducts in approximately 30% of cases. In the biliary tree the procedure is useful in identifying retained bile duct calculi and stenoses from neoplasm, inflammation or post surgical fibrosis.

Technique

The endoscopic examination of stomach and duodenum, and the catheterization of the ampulla is performed by a trained endoscopist. Description of the technique is outside the scope of this book. It is usually the function of the radiologist to ensure that optimal radiographs are taken and that they are correctly interpreted.

It is usual to take 30 × 24 cm spot films of the distal common bile duct, common hepatic duct, the intrahepatic ducts and the entire length of the pancreatic duct. A most important final film is the erect drainage film where the patient is turned from a prone to a supine position and the table head raised 45°. This view is useful in separating air bubbles from calculi. Air bubbles will float upwards while calculi will sink to the bottom of the bile duct.

BILIARY CALCULUS EXTRACTION

Indications

1. Calculi in the biliary tree shown at post cholecystectomy T-tube cholangiography, may be removed through the T-tube track.
2. The maximum diameter of a calculus likely to be removed through such a track is 1 cm. Larger calculi may sometimes be crushed in the bile duct, and removed in pieces.
3. The optimum time for performing the procedure is 6 weeks after operation. This allows sufficient time for a well defined fibrous track to form around the T-tube, to allow manipulation of the extraction catheter.

Patient preparation

1. The patient must be premedicated with an antibiotic. A suitable regimen is Gentamycin 80 mg and Ampicillin 500 mg both IM and given one hour before the procedure.
2. No fasting is necessary.
3. Since the procedure is often uncomfortable it is wise to give a suitable analgesic before beginning.

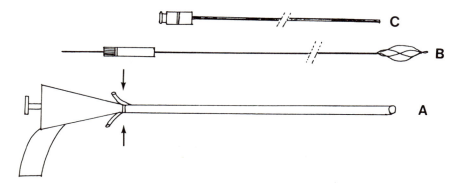

Fig. 3.7 Typical biliary calculus extraction set. (A) steerable wide bore catheter with side branches for injection of contrast and insertion of basket and sheath catheter (arrows). (B) An 0.89 mm (0.035 in) wire with collapsable basket which fits inside. (C) sheath catheter.

Equipment (Fig. 3.7)

Several calculus removal systems are available commercially but the basic features common to all are:
1. An outer wide bore 8 or 13F steerable catheter, through which contrast medium can be injected and finer wires and catheters can be passed.
2. An 0.89 mm (0.035 in) bore sheath catheter over an 0.89 mm (0.035 in) wire which terminates in a collapsable wire basket (Dormia basket).

Technique

1. An initial T-tube cholangiogram is performed to identify the position of calculi.
2. The T-tube is removed.
3. The steerable wide catheter, with the Dormia basket closed inside its own sheath and advanced half way along the steerable catheter, is filled with contrast to expel air bubbles.
4. The steerable catheter, with the closed Dormia basket inside, is advanced along the T-tube track under fluoroscopic control and turned up or down the bile duct to where the calculus lies.
5. The Dormia basket, still closed inside its sheath is now advanced beyond the calculus.
6. The Dormia basket is opened by advancing it out of its sheath.
7. The calculus is manoeuvred into the basket which is closed around it by withdrawing the wire tail of the basket into its sheath.
8. The whole assembly including the calculus is removed.

Practical problems

The foregoing is a simplified version of what is sometimes a very difficult procedure.

1. Inability to engage the stone in the basket. A useful move is to push the basket to and fro with a rapid jiggling motion close by the calculus. This often has the effect of snaring it. It may be useful to move the stone to a relatively fixed position such as the distal common bile duct or into the orifice of the T-tube track. With the calculus thus fixed it may be possible to engage it in the basket.

2. The stone is too big for the basket. In this case the stone will have to be broken up either by repeatedly punching it with the wire end of the basket, or by engaging one part of it in the basket in order to break off a portion when the basket is closed.

3. Inability to get the stone and basket back along the T-tube track. If the stone is only a little wider than the track this can be enlarged with the aid of nephrostomy dilators to a suitable calibre. The dilatation should be performed alongside the basket wire with the outer steerable catheter removed.

Post procedure care

1. If the extraction has gone smoothly and the operator is sure no calculi are left, the T-tube track can be left to close over.
2. If there has been manipulation of the ampullary region of the duct, oedema and spasm may result in temporary biliary obstruction. To avoid this it is wise to leave a 10 French soft rubber catheter in the bile duct and draining to the exterior.
3. A catheter should also be left in situ if there is any suggestion that calculi still remain. This will allow a check cholangiogram the following day.

PERCUTANEOUS TRANSHEPATIC CHOLANGIOGRAPHY

With the introduction of the Chiba University or 'Skinny' needle, percutaneous transhepatic cholangiography has become a safe and easily performed procedure. The success rate should be 95% for obstructive and 85% for non-obstructive lesions.

Indications

1. To determine the cause of obstructive jaundice.
2. Post-operative jaundice considered likely to be caused by stricture or calculus in the bile ducts.
3. To determine the cause of recurrent jaundice, for example to distinguish between primary biliary cirrhosis, sclerosing cholangitis and recurrent infective cholangitis, when laboratory studies have not been helpful.
4. As a prelude to a percutaneous drainage procedure.

Equipment

1. 23 gauge thin wall Chiba needle, sterile drapes and skin cleanser.
2. Local anaesthetic.
3. Water soluble contrast, e.g. diatrizoate (Hypaque 60% or Urografin 60%).

Patient preparation

1. The clotting time is checked and corrected if necessary.
2. Routine cover with antibiotics is advisable. A suitable regime is ampicillin 500 mg IM and Gentamicin 80 mg IM both 1 hour before the procedure.

Technique

The patient is placed supine on a fluoroscopic table. The injection point is selected with fluoroscopy. Generally, this is the tenth or eleventh intercostal space, 3 cm anterior to the mid-axillary line. The entry site selected should be seen on fluoroscopy to be below the costophrenic angle on deep inspiration and to be generally opposite the bulk of the liver mass.

The skin is swabbed and draped in sterile fashion. Local anaesthetic is infiltrated along the projected needle track down to the peritoneum. The Chiba needle is now inserted horizontally in suspended respiration, until the tip lies at a point midway between the rib cage and vertebral column. Normal respiration is resumed and a flexible polyethylene tube and a syringe of contrast medium are attached.

Small amounts of contrast are injected as the needle is slowly withdrawn. Once the bile ducts have been entered they are easily seen and should then be filled with more contrast medium. Contrast injected interstitially tends to stay localized in a pool, and when the portal veins are entered it quickly flows away from the needle tip.

Bile is aspirated, if possible, to facilitate filling the biliary tree with contrast without overdistension. In many cases, however, no bile can be aspirated, usually because a very small biliary radicle has been entered. The amount of contrast medium required to outline the biliary tree is variable, but may be up to 50 ml. Mixing of contrast with bile may be facilitated by tipping the table until the patient is erect, subsequently positioning prone and on each side.

Radiographs of the entire biliary system are taken AP lateral and 45° oblique to right and left, coned views of the distal end of the bile duct are also taken.

Difficulties and complications

1. Bile peritonitis. This occurs infrequently with a fine gauge needle and the procedure no longer needs to be scheduled pre-operatively. However, care should be taken to puncture the biliary tree in the liver, for an extra hepatic puncture may lead to a significant leak.

2. Intraperitoneal bleeding. This is not usually a serious problem in a patient with a normal clotting profile.

3. Cholangitis. This may occur if the biliary tree is overdistended, in spite of antibiotic cover.

4. Pain. This may result from subcapsular contrast. It is not a serious problem and is easily managed with analgesics.

Failure to enter the biliary tree

If no radicle can be entered on the first pass, a slightly different angle should be selected, preferably without withdrawing the needle tip from the liver, and the procedure repeated. The number of separate passes is limited by clinical discretion, keeping in mind that the greater the number of capsular punctures the greater the complication rate.

Failure to visualize the entire biliary tree

In this case the contrast may merely be localized in one part of the biliary system. The needle should be removed, and the patient rolled to lateral and prone positions before the films are taken.

The films obtained should be closely examined to ensure that both the right and left duct systems have been outlined. Non-filling of the left duct system is a particular problem with obstructing tumours around the common hepatic duct. If the left duct is blocked by a benign stenosis of long standing, the left lobe of the liver may be atrophic; a fact of great significance to a treating surgeon. A second pass with the Chiba needle may be required to outline the left hepatic duct branches.

Percutaneous biliary drainage

In patients with obstruction of the biliary tree demonstrated on PTC or ultrasound, temporary or permanent drainage, either to the skin or duodenum, may be achieved by placement of a large bore catheter through the obstruction. Pre-operative decompression and relief of jaundice is useful in reducing the high operative risk of renal failure in the severely jaundiced patient. It is also possible to leave an indwelling stent in situ, without the need for a percutaneous component.

Equipment

1. 1 × Surgimed-type 6F splenoportogram needle.
2. 7F, 8F and 10F dilators.
3. 1 × 0.047 in broad J guidewire.
4. 1 × 8.3F pigtail biliary drainage catheter.

Technique

1. The patient is prepared as for a PTC which is done first to outline the biliary tree.
2. Under fluoroscopic control, with lateral and AP screening, a Surgimed-type splenoportogram 6F needle is inserted through a small skin incision at the same site as for PTC. The needle is advanced toward a large centrally placed intrahepatic bile duct. Once a free flow of bile is obtained, an 0.047 in broad J guidewire is advanced through the Surgimed sheath through the stenosis into the duodenum. The sheath is then removed and the track is progressively dilated by passing a series

Fig. 3.8 (opposite) Percutaneous biliary drainage with indwelling stent placement. (A) The dilated biliary tree, previously opacified by PTC, is punctured with a wide bore needle. (B) A wire is passed through the needle, manoeuvred through an obstructing tumour of the bile duct and into the duodenum. (C) After track dilatation a stent is advanced over the wire by a pusher tube. When the stent placement is optimal, the wire and pusher tube are removed.

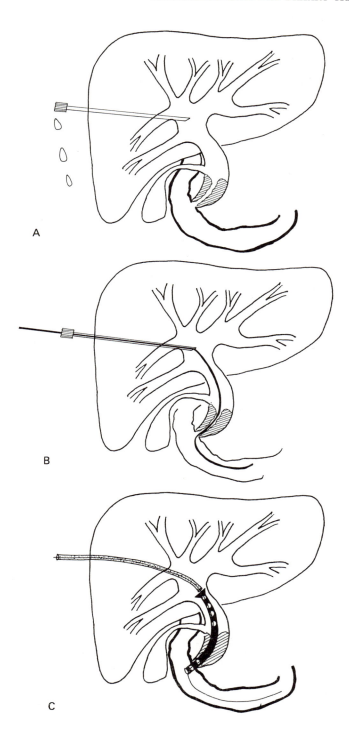

A

B

C

of dilators up to 10F over the guidewire. An 8.3F pigtail biliary drainage catheter is then passed over the guidewire until its tip is coiled in the duodenum.

Once satisfactory drainage is established, the catheter is fixed by suture and plastic disc to the skin. The catheter is left draining into a skin bag for 48 hours. After this it may be sealed, leading to internal drainage. Post operatively the catheter should be flushed with saline daily to prevent clogging with debris.

Problems

1. If the catheter cannot be negotiated past the obstruction, a straight drain tube may be left in an intrahepatic duct with external drainage. It is often worth a second attempt at negotiating an obstruction after 24 hours. The oedema from the first attempt may then be less and perhaps more importantly the operator will be fresh.
2. Copious blood comes back along the splenoportogram needle. In this case the needle is likely to have punctured a portal vein branch. If the bleeding does not stop once the needle is withdrawn a little, the entry track may need to be occluded with Gelfoam plugs to avoid haemoperitoneum.

Indwelling stents

These offer considerable advantages over external biliary catheters and should be used whenever possible. Several companies make stent kits.

Technique

The procedure is exactly as for insertion of an external drainage catheter except that a long guide catheter is passed over the guidewire instead of an external drain tube. This guide catheter is passed through into the duodenum. The stent is so constructed to fit over the guide catheter. The stent is advanced into the correct position across the obstruction by means of a pusher tube also over the guide catheter. When the stent is judged to be correctly placed, the pusher tube and the inner guide catheter are withdrawn and the stent is left in situ.

FURTHER READING

Anacker H, Weiss H D, Kramann B, Rupp N 1974 Experience with endoscopic retrograde pancreatography. American Journal of Roentgenology 122: 375–384

Baker H L Jr, Hodgson J R 1960 Further studies on the accuracy of oral cholecystography. Radiology 74: 239–245

Bean W J, Smith S L, Mahorner H R 1973 Equipment for non operative removal of biliary tract stones. Radiology 107: 452–453

Bean W J, Smith S, Calonje M A 1974 Percutaneous removal of residual biliary tract stones: problems encountered in a series of 44 cases. Radiology 113: 1–9

Bean W J, Smith S, Calonje M A 1975 T-tube tract dilatation for removal of large biliary stones. Radiology 115: 485–486

Bree R L, Flynn R E 1972 Hypotonic duodenography in the evaluation of choledocholithiasis and obstructive jaundice. American Journal of Roentgenology 116: 309–319

Buonocore E 1976 Transhepatic percutaneous cholangiography. Radiologic Clinics of North America 14: 527–542

Burcharth F, Jensen L I, Olesen K 1979 Endoprosthesis for internal drainage of the biliary tract. Gastroenterology 77: 133–137

Burgener F A 1980 Intravenous cholangiography: experimental evaluation of the time–density–retention concept. American Journal of Radiology 134: 665–667

Dooley J S, Dick R, Irving D, Olney J, Sherlock S 1981 Relief of bile duct obstruction by the percutaneous transhepatic insertion of an endoprosthesis. Clinical Radiology 32: 163–172

Ekberg O 1977 Double contrast examination of the small bowel. Gastrointestinal Radiology 1 (No. 4) 349–353

Evers K, Laufer I, Gordon R L, Kressel H Y, Herlinger H, Gohel V K 1981 Double contrast enema examination for detection of rectal carcinoma. Radiology 140: 635–639

Freeny P C, Bilbao M K, Raton R M 1976 Blind evaluation of endoscopic retrograde cholangio pancreatography in the diagnosis of pancreatic carcinoma: the 'double duct' and other signs. Radiology 119: 271–274

Gelfand D W 1976 Double contrast examination of the gastrointestinal tract: the Japanese style double contrast examination of the stomach. Gastrointestinal Radiology 1: 7–17

Gelfand D W 1978 High density, low viscosity barium for five mucosal detail on double contrast upper gastrointestinal examinations. American Journal of Roentgenology 130: 831–833

Gelfand D W, Ott D J 1982 Barium sulphate suspensions: an evaluation of available products. American Journal of Roentgenology 138: 935–941

Gohel V K, Kressel H Y, Laufer I 1978 Double contrast artefacts. Gastrointestinal Radiology 3: 139–146

Goldsmith M R, Paul R E, Poplack W E, Moore J P, Matsue H, Bloom S 1976 Evaluation of routine double contrast views of the anterior wall of the stomach. American Journal of Roentgenology 126: 1159–1163

Goldstein H M, Dodd G D 1976 Double contrast examination of the oesophagus. Gastrointestinal Radiology 1: 3–6

Herlinger H 1978 A modified technique for the double contrast small bowel enema. Gastrointestinal Radiology 3 (No. 2) 201–207

Hodgson J R 1970 The technical aspects of cholecystography. Radiologic Clinics of North America 8: 85–97

Kelvin F M, Gardner R, Vas W, Stephenson G W 1981 Colorectal carcinoma missed on double contrast barium enema: a problem in perception. Amercial Journal of Roentgenology 137: 307–313

Laufer I 1982 Radiology of esophagitis. Radiologic Clinics of North America 20: 687–699

Mahorner H R, Bean W J 1971 Removal of a residual stone from the common bile duct without surgery. Annals of Surgery 173: 857–860

Miller R E, Maglinte D 1982 Barium pneumocolon: technologist performed '7 pump' method. Amercial Journal of Roentgenology 139: 1230–1232

Miller R E, Sellink J L 1979 Enteroclysis: the small bowel enema: how to succeed and how to fail. Gastrointestinal Radiology 4 (No. 3) 269–283

Miller R E, Chernish S M, Rosenak B D, Rodda B E 1973 Hypotonic duodenography with glucagon. Radiology 108: 35–42

Montgomery D P, Clamp S E, de Dombal P T et al 1982 A comparison of barium sulphate preparations used for the double contrast barium meal. Clinical Radiology 33: 265–269

Nolan D J, Cadman P J 1987 The small bowel enema made easy. Clinical Radiology 38: 295–301

Poplack W, Paul R E, Goldsmith M, Matsue H, Moore J P, Norton R 1975 Demonstration of erosive gastritis by the double contrast technique. Radiology 117: 519–521

Press A J 1975 Practical significance of gastric rugal folds. American Journal of Roentgenology 125: 172–183

Rabinor K R, MacArthur J 1976 A simple technique for performing intraoperative cholangiography. Archives of Surgery 111: 608

Samuel E 1959 Operative cholangiography. British Journal of Radiology 32: 669–672

Scholz F J, Johnson D O, Wise R E 1975 Intravenous cholangiography — optimum dosage and methodology. Radiology 114: 513–518

Silvis S E, Rohrmann C A, Vennes J A 1973 Diagnostic criteria for evaluation of the endoscopic pancreatogram. Gastrointestinal Endoscopy 20: 51–55

Tabrisky J, Lindstrom R L, Hanelin L G, Pfisterer W F 1976 Chiba percutaneous transhepatic cholangiography. American Journal of Roentgenology 126: 755–760

4

Vascular radiology

INTRODUCTION

Every angiographer has his or her particular preferences with regard to the needles, wire guide and catheter used in routine procedures. This manual is not intended to be exhaustive and some procedures which are not in regular use at The Royal Melbourne Hospital have been excluded. The items specified and methods described in this chapter are those in use at The Royal Melbourne Hospital. Alternative items may be substituted to suit the reader's preference. Digital subtraction angiography allows the use of smaller catheter diameters and less concentration of contrast than specified below.

Patient selection

Patients with very small arteries, severe atherosclerosis, and diabetes are at increased risk of complications. In such cases alternative methods such as digital subtraction angiography or computed tomography should be considered. In the final analysis it is the radiologist who must decide if a particular procedure is warranted as he or she is responsible for any complications. There is no place in angiography for unnecessary catheterization and contrast injection.

PATIENT PREPARATION

Since vascular radiology is by its nature invasive, it is associated with a small but significant morbidity and for this reason informed consent should always be obtained prior to the procedure. This consent should be obtained by the radiologist who will perform the procedure and where possible this consent should be obtained prior to the arrival of the patient in the angiographic department.

In most patients no preparation is required beyond restriction of solid food for 4 hours prior to the procedure while allowing free oral fluids. In anxious patients oral diazepam is effective if given in 10 mg dose one hour before the examination. Alternatively an intramuscular or intravenous opiate, an antiemetic and diazepam can be used. Atropine (0.6 mg) is given intravenously if a vaso-vagal attack occurs. However, if the procedure is painful or very long or the patient is uncooperative then a neurolept or general anaesthesia should be used.

Because neurological observations are made routinely during neuroangiography, sedation is not given unless the radiologist considers it is absolutely necessary.

The access site must be cleared of hair and thoroughly washed with an antiseptic, preferably one containing alcohol. Infection at the puncture site is fortunately rare. However, in our experience, hair emboli have been seen in the carotid arteries following femoral artery puncture on two occasions (Tress & Field 1981).

An adhesive skin drape is convenient if the patient will be moved during the examination. The drapes should be large enough to prevent soiling of the wire guides during catheter changes and cover the upper sides of the examination table.

Long and involved cases may require a urinary catheter and an IV line to both drain urine and maintain fluid balance. A full bladder, a hard examination table and a long procedure can be a most uncomfortable experience.

METHOD OF ACCESS TO THE CIRCULATION

Arterial puncture

Femoral artery

Retrograde access. Arterial access is readily available in the groin (common femoral artery), and in almost all cases this is the access site used. The puncture must be made in a site at which the artery can be compressed by the fingers both proximal to and distal to the puncture. This means below the inguinal ligament. Failure to observe this precaution has caused fatal haemorrhage. For retrograde aortic catheterization the usual puncture is made at or below the skin crease in the groin (see Fig. 4.1). The artery is palpated and a total of 5–10 ml of local anaesthetic (1% xylocaine) injected very slowly around the intended puncture site avoiding injection into the artery itself. Rapid injection of local anaesthetic is very painful for the patient. With a No. 11 scalpel blade an incision is made in the skin no bigger than the diameter of the catheter to be used. An arterial puncture needle is advanced bevel upwards gently through the skin in an angle of about 50° towards the artery until pulsation is felt at the tip of the needle. Since only the front wall should be punctured a single-part needle (Cook SDN 18–7) is preferred. Further advancement of the needle results in entry to the lumen and a free flow of blood. A 'J-tip' wire guide (Cook TSCF 1.5 Sachs 145) is inserted through the needle and up the artery for several centimetres (see Fig. 4.2). There should be no sensation of resistance to the

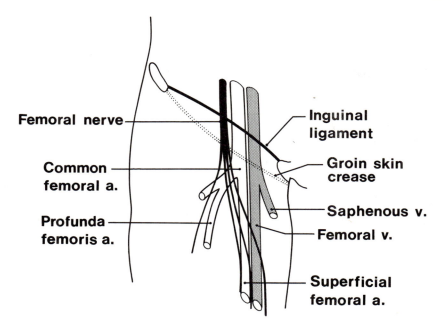

Fig. 4.1 *Anatomy of the femoral triangle.*
A schematic diagram showing the major vessels at the groin. Note the relationship between the groin skin crease and the inguinal ligament.

passage of the wire guide. If there is resistance further advancement should only be performed under fluoroscopic control. In the event fluoroscopy is recommended for wire guide insertion of more than a few centimetres. When the wire guide is in a satisfactory position the needle is removed over the wire and the artery compressed with the fingers. It is useful to develop the ability to compress the artery with two or three fingers and hold the wire guide firmly with the thumb and index finger. The assistant then wipes the wire guide clean with a wet gauze pad and feeds the catheter over the wire guide towards the operator until the wire guide appears at the hub end of the catheter. The assistant holds the wire guide taut without pulling it out of the artery (which is why the operator holds on to the wire guide) and feeds the catheter up to the puncture site. The catheter is then inserted into the artery over the wire guide with a slight rotary motion. Generally the assistant holds the wire guide so that it is not advanced further as the catheter enters the artery. When the catheter is in the desired position the wire guide is removed and the catheter is aspirated and then flushed with heparinized normal saline. The aspiration and flushing is best performed using two separate syringes; one for the aspiration, and another filled with heparinized saline for flushing, to avoid any blood clot emboli. The wire guide is then carefully cleaned and placed ready for further use.

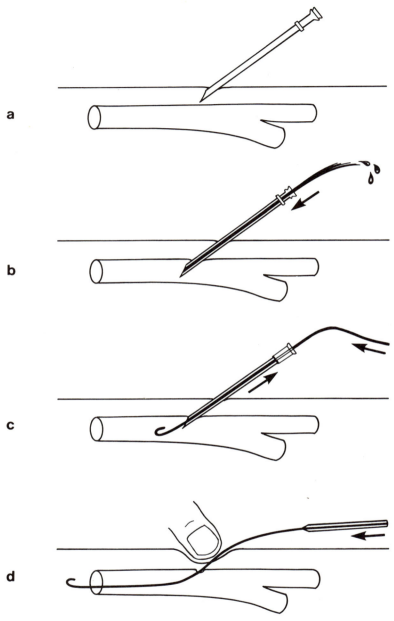

Fig. 4.2 *Technique of arterial puncture with single part needle.*
(a) The needle is advanced bevel uppermost down to the artery at an oblique angle. Arterial pulsations are transmitted along the needle when it comes in contact with the arterial wall.
(b) The needle is advanced until a spurt of blood appears from the needle. (c) A safety wire guide is advanced up the needle and well up the artery. (d) The needle has been removed and finger pressure is used to compress the puncture site while a catheter is advanced along the wire guide and into the artery.

Antegrade access. If the catheter is to be passed in antegrade fashion down the superficial artery then the puncture in the skin is usually at or above the inguinal ligament but because of the oblique path of the needle the arterial puncture is still below the ligament.

The common femoral artery is palpated at the inguinal ligament and local anaesthetic infiltrated around the artery about 1–2 cm below the ligament. The artery is punctured with a SDN needle and a 1.5 mm 'J-tip' wire guide inserted down the artery for several centimetres or until resistance is felt. A 5F catheter is curved at its tip with hot water and inserted over the wire guide into the artery. The wire guide is removed, the catheter flushed, and contrast medium (Iopamiro 300) injected gently under fluoroscopic control. If the catheter is in the profunda femoris then it is withdrawn under fluoroscopy and the tip rotated until it is directed towards the superficial femoral artery. The wire guide and catheter are then advanced down the artery to the desired position. This technique requires puncture above the common femoral bifurcation. Turning the patient into the opposite posterior oblique will open the common femoral bifurcation.

If the bifurcation is very high the superficial femoral artery can be punctured directly. This can be done without removing a catheter already below the bifurcation which has entered the profunda femoris artery.

Direct puncture of the carotid artery

As most carotid artery punctures are made for carotid angiography a wire guide is generally not inserted. The needle is stabilized with wet gauze strips and a short connecting tube attached for the injection of contrast and flushing saline. It is good practice to aspirate gently and flush the needle continuously to ensure that the tip of the needle does not become subintimal and cause an occluding dissection of the wall. Some needle sets have a short wire guide on the end of a cannula to allow advancement of the needle but we have not routinely used them.

Direct puncture of any of the superficial arteries has been described elsewhere (Greitz & Lindgren 1971, Johnsrube & Jackson 1979).

Brachial artery ('axillary')

The brachial artery can be punctured in the upper third of the arm as a safer alternative to axillary puncture. The artery is easily palpated and compressed against the head of the humerus when the arm is flexed at the elbow, abducted at the shoulder and the hand placed palm uppermost under the head (see Fig. 4.3). Access to the descending aorta is easier from the left side and as most people are right handed the dominant hand is not at risk from left sided punctures. For a right-handed operator the left side is also easier to approach. The complication rate is higher with

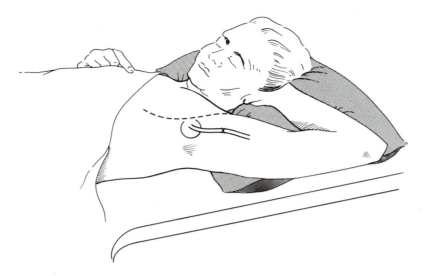

Fig. 4.3 *Patient position for 'axilliary' artery puncture.*
The patient is positioned with the arm abducted and the hand placed palm uppermost under the head. The brachial artery rather than the axillary artery is punctured (X). The axillary artery is hard to palpate or compress above the head of the humerus.

brachial or axillary punctures (Johnsrube & Jackson 1979) and they are only used when a femoral approach is contraindicated or impossible.

A small volume of local anaesthetic is used because of the possibility of producing an unwanted partial brachial plexus block and the fluid may make the artery hard to feel. The artery is punctured and a 1.5 mm 'J-tip' wire guide advanced well into the ascending aorta. A 6.5F catheter with a long recurved tip (SIM2L Cook BPS) is inserted into the ascending aorta and the curve formed on the aortic valve. Avoid entering the left ventricle and withdraw the catheter or wire guide if necessary. For the lower aortic catheterization the catheter with wire guide in situ is withdrawn until the catheter tip is directed towards the descending aorta and the wire guide advanced down the aorta (see Fig. 4.4). The recurved tip of the catheter allows catheterization of any of the arch vessels from either axillary artery. Selective catheterization is generally limited to the length of the recurved tip.

After the procedure the radial pulse should be palpable while the bleeding point is compressed. As a result of the local anaesthetic, proprioception may be impaired in the arm for several hours after the angiography the patient is advised against using the affected arm until sensation in the fingers is normal. A change in colour or onset of pain in the hand after the procedure is to be reported to the radiologist immediately as a late occlusion of the artery may have occurred.

The major cause of brachial plexus injury is pressure from a haematoma in or around the neurovascular bundle.

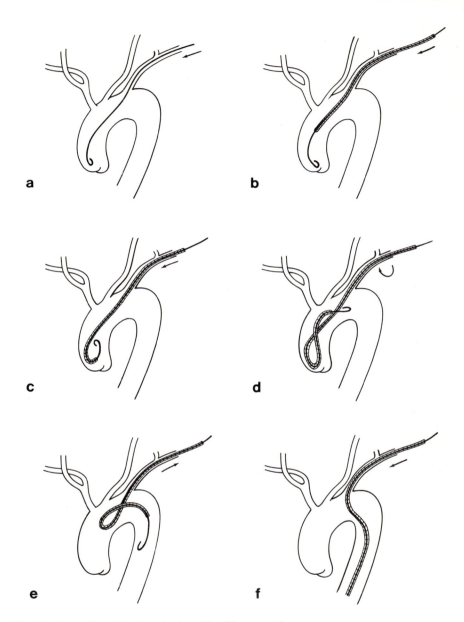

Fig. 4.4 *Antegrade aortic catheterization with a Simmons catheter.*
(a) Via the left brachial artery a wire guide is advanced to the ascending aorta. (b) The catheter is introduced over the wire guide. (c) The wire guide is reflected upwards from the aortic sinus to allow reformation of the loop in the catheter. (d) The catheter is advanced with slight rotation and the Simmons loop is formed in the ascending aorta with the wire guide at the origin of the descending aorta. (e) Traction on the catheter will advance the catheter and wire guide into the descending aorta. (f) The wire guide and catheter are advanced down to the desired level in the thoracic or abdominal aorta.

Translumbar aortography

This method is usually performed with a needle technique for the diagnosis of aorto-iliac and femoral disease. The needle we recommend has a closed end and one side hole close to the tip opposite the bevel (see Fig. 4.5).

Translumbar puncture can be performed either below or above the level of the renal arteries. In practice almost every portion and branch of the abdominal aorta has been punctured in this way. In our opinion the puncture should be high enough to demonstrate the status of the renal arteries as well as the lower aorta.

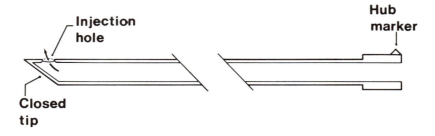

Fig. 4.5 *The RMH translumbar needle.*
This 18 gauge needle has a closed tip and a single side hole near the tip. The hub marker indicates the position of the side hole.

The patient is laid prone on the examination table and a point marked which is roughly one hand-breadth above the iliac crest and a similar distance lateral to the lumbar spinous processes (see Fig. 4.6). In small patients this is almost at the lower border of the twelfth rib. The skin is prepared with antiseptic solution and the area draped as for any angiogram. Local anaesthetic is injected into the skin and superficial muscles. For a high puncture the needle is directed towards the twelfth thoracic vertebral body but for a low puncture the needle is directed at right angles to the spine. Purists scorn the use of fluoroscopy but the aorta is often calcified or tortuous and fluoroscopic guidance is often useful. The needle is advanced obliquely towards the anterior third of the vertebral body, and after the resistance of the vertebra is felt, the needle is withdrawn slightly and angled more anteriorly. With further advancement the pulsation of the aorta can be felt transmitted by the needle. A short jab is usually enough to place the tip of the needle within the aortic lumen. A flexible tube is attached and contrast injected gently to confirm a satisfactory placement of the needle within the lumen of the aorta. Provided the aorta fills well without intimal straining with contrast, and a low injection rate is used, then puncture of a branch can be accepted. If fluoroscopy has not been used the position of the needle will only become apparent when the films are examined.

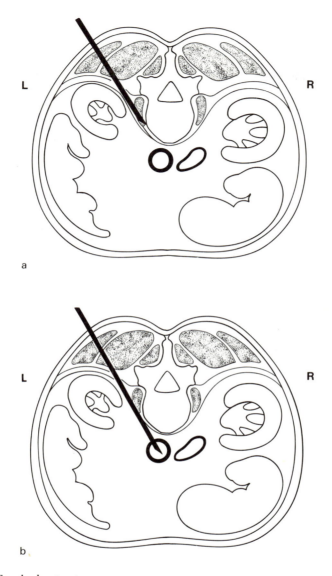

Fig. 4.6 *Translumbar puncture.*
(a) The needle is inserted between the kidney and the vertebral body. If the needle strikes the vertebra it is withdrawn slightly and angled more vertically. (b) When pulsation of the aorta is felt on the needle, it is advanced about 1 cm or until blood flows freely from the needle.

Although catheterization of the aorta has been reported from this approach it is not a technique for the occasional operator and the risk of bleeding after the catheterization is significant.

Surgical exposure

This method is usually performed by cardiologists who cut down on the brachial artery and perform an arteriotomy above the elbow for access for cardiac catheterization. It has not been necessary in our angiographic suite for cardiac or other angiography. Formal training in arterial suture is required to avoid loss of the brachial or radial artery pulse following the procedure.

Venous catheterization

The arm veins are easily accessible to percutaneous methods and the femoral vein is also easy to puncture as it lies medial to the femoral artery in the femoral triangle. The best puncture site for femoral veins is near the apex of the femoral triangle. A 10 ml syringe is attached to an arterial needle and aspirated gently as the needle is withdrawn. It is not necessary to have the patient hold their breath or perform a Valsalva manoeuvre. A guide is advanced as for the femoral artery and exchanged for a catheter in the usual way.

CHOICE OF CATHETER AND WIRE GUIDE

Catheter

Diameter

In general terms the smallest diameter catheter within the constraints of the flow rate required should be used as this lessens the chance of damage to the arterial wall and minimizes the length of time 'wasted' compressing the puncture site after the procedure. Unfortunately some small diameter high flow catheters are stiff or kink rather easily.

Material

For most purposes polyethylene tubing is satisfactory but polyurethane and other materials such as woven Dacron are available. A catheter with a wire braded wall offers much greater torque and predictable control than non-braded materials but for the bulk of angiography braded catheters are an unnecessary expense for one-time use.

Reuse of catheters is unsatisfactory as the characteristics manufactured into the catheter cannot be guaranteed after sterilization and the total removal of all pyrogens is almost impossible. Certainly in our hospital it is no longer economic in terms of the time and staff involved in cleaning or the possibility of litigation if a 'one-time use only' product is reused.

Wire guide

A wire guide is a precision instrument which is often subjected to considerable stress during a difficult catheterization. Blood products are always found inside the spring coils and after cleaning corrosion will be seen if the wire guide is pulled apart and inspected. The Teflon coating of re-cycled wires may flake off the wire guide during cleaning or on the passage through the needle. The temperature of most hospital-based sterilizing systems is sufficient to impart a memory of the coils in the wire guide which may make it act in a different way to that intended by its manufacturer.

The remarks made above with respect to reuse of catheters apply more firmly to wire guides.

A wire guide should contain a safety core which is welded to the tip to prevent loss of the tip should the wire fracture. In some of the situations described later in this chapter use of other wire guides without this feature could be hazardous.

The choice of a particular shape and tip configuration of a wire guide is a matter of personal preference and the types described are those in use at The Royal Melbourne Hospital. For vascular work all the wire guides are Teflon coated to minimize friction in the catheter and build-up of thrombus on the wire guide.

The smallest diameter 'J' tip (1.5 mm curve) is used for all aortic catheterizations and a 10 cm floppy tip with tapered mandrel (Newton) is used for almost all selective and sub-selective catheterizations.

To make ordering easier a full range of wire guides is only kept in one size which in our case is 0.89 mm (0.035 in) diameter and 145 cm in length. A limited stock of other sizes is kept for special situations. The indications for the use of these are discussed later in this chapter.

CHOICE OF CONTRAST MEDIA

Available iodinated radiographic contrast media fall into two main types; ionic (standard) contrast media and the newer non-ionic contrast media (see Fig. 4.7).

Non-ionic contrast media (Iopamiro) are less toxic on the intima and vital organs than ionic media but at present they are much more expensive. From the patient's point of view non-ionic media are much more pleasant as there is almost no sensation of heat as with the ionic media (Kallenbauge & Praestholm 1982). In patients in whom the total dose of contrast is a limiting factor then non-ionic media are to be preferred because of their lower osmolality.

For cerebral angiography ionic contrast should contain no sodium ions. The contrast used at The Royal Melbourne Hospital for cerebral and spinal angiography is Angiografin (Schering) which is a pure meglumine diatrizoate. This contrast is also used for peripheral angiography when it is mixed

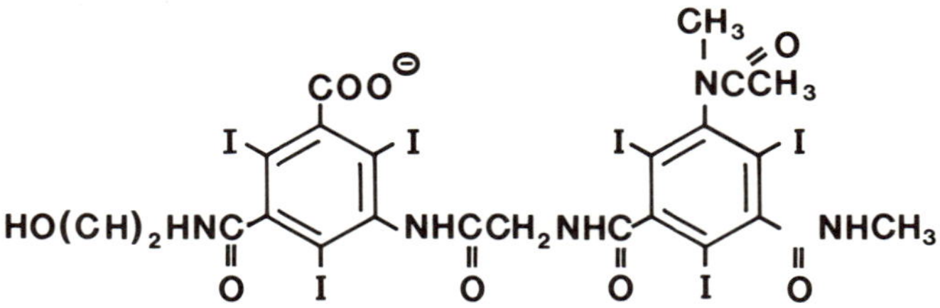

IOXAGLATE

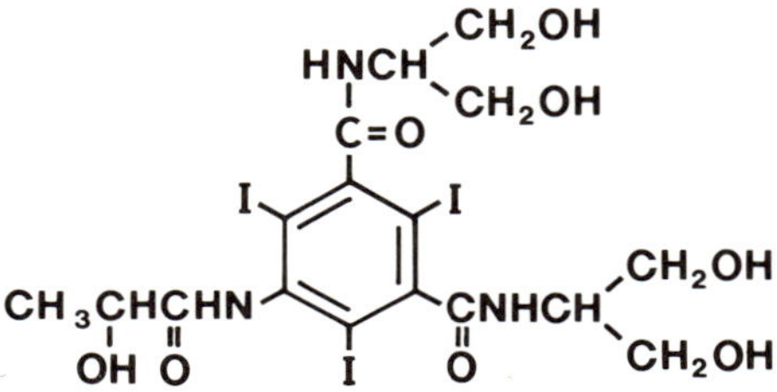

IOPAMIDOL

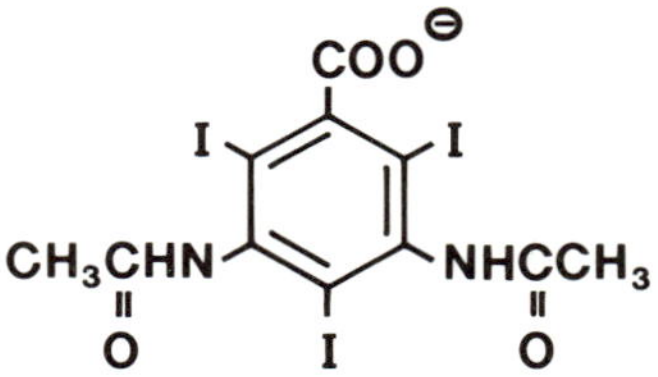

DIATRIZOATE

Fig. 4.7 *Intravascular contrast media formulae.*
Standard formulae for an hypertonic ionic contrast (Diatrizoate), a low osmolar ionic contrast (Ioxaglate) and a low osmolar non-ionic contrast (Iopamidol). Note the large number of hydroxyl and oxygen groups in Iopamidol compared to Diatrizoate.

with 1% xylocaine in a ratio of 1 of xylocaine to 7 of Angiografin by volume to minimize patient discomfort. For cardiac angiography ionic contrast should contain roughly isotonic amounts of sodium ions (Fischer & Thomson 1978). Iopamiro 370 (Schering) is used for all cardiac angiography, digital subtraction angiography and aortography (except aorto-femoral aortograms) at The Royal Melbourne Hospital.

Cerebral angiography with sodium-containing iodinated contrast media has been shown to damage the cerebral blood–brain barrier (Sage et al 1981).

The choice of contrast media is determined by many factors including cost and reliability of supply but the incidence of toxic and allergic reactions should also be considered and our experience with Angiografin and Urografin has shown a very low incidence of contrast-related reactions. In the future if the price is reduced a single non-ionic contrast medium could be used for all angiography (and myelography).

COMPLICATIONS

In even the best angiography units the overall complication rate is about 3% or less depending to some extent on the type of patients being examined (Sigstedt & Lunderquist 1978). While in some cases the cause and effect are clear, in many instances the complication is only presumed to be as a direct result of the catheterization.

Catheter complications

Most of the complications are the result of damage to the blood vessel wall by the catheter or wire guide or follow the inadverdent injection of air of particulate matter through the catheter. Haematoma formation at the puncture site is fairly common but usually not serious. False aneurysm may complicate any arterial puncture but particularly in calcified arteries or after the use of very large catheters. Rarely, suture of the puncture may be required to control the bleeding.

Occlusion of the artery may occur if the intima is stripped or otherwise damaged. Occlusion is more likely to occur if the flow is in the same direction as the dissection. For this reason a dissection in the iliac artery may go unnoticed but a carotid dissection is usually the cause of occlusion of the artery.

Emboli should be entirely preventable. The recipient organ determines the severity of the complication. An air bubble in the internal carotid will cause a cerebral ischaemic episode which may or may not resolve whereas a similar air bubble in the coronary circulation is often unnoticed until the cine film is developed. The dissection of the internal carotid in an otherwise healthy young adult is often not as disastrous as a similar occlusion in a patient with diseased carotid arteries.

Avoidance of complications requires a meticulous technique and competent operators including the radiographer, nurse and radiologist as in some cases the extra time taken to perform the examination may be the underlying cause of the complication. Catheter and wire guide manipulation require a combination of touch and vision to minimize damage to the vessel. Even a flexible wire guide in some hands is a lethal weapon.

Within the circulation after about 15 minutes the catheter is coated inside and out with a film of adherent platelets and blood products. The use of systemic heparin has been shown to reduce substantially the complication rate in coronary angiography (Adams et al 1973). Most non-cardiac angiography is performed without systemic heparin but the catheters are flushed much more frequently with a heparinized solution. As a rule of thumb a wire guide should be removed and wiped after 2 minutes use and the catheter aspirated and then flushed using separate syringes at the same interval.

Fracture of the catheter or wire guide is a rare cause of complications if the Seldinger technique is used. Most of the fragments lost in the circulation are the result of the use of needle–catheter combinations. With single use of wire guides containing a safety wire we have not lost a section of wire guide in the circulation even though the wire guide has on occasion fractured after very heavy use or purposeful bending.

CONTRAST MEDIA REACTIONS

Reactions to contrast media may be considered as pathophysiological effects or idiosyncratic (anaphylactoid) reactions.

The pathophysiological effects are consequent upon the high osmolarity of the compound, the presence of single valence cations, and the inherent molecular toxicity of the compound. These include changes in blood pressure, heart rate, cardiac output and subjective feeling of heat or pain. Neurotoxicity, altered renal function, erythrocyte deformity, and endothelial damage may also occur. These effects are reduced when a non-ionic contrast is used but not by the administration of antihistamines or corticosteroids.

Idiosyncratic reactions are manifest by urticaria, angioneurotic oedema, bronchospasm, respiratory arrest and vasomotor collapse. Generally these reactions are reduced by premedication with antihistamines and corticosteroids or by treatment with adrenaline.

The chance of contrast medium reaction is about 6 per 10 000 (Shehadi & Toniolo 1980) but this increases significantly if there is a history of atopia or prior contrast reaction. Skin testing is of little use as the reactions are not IgE-mediated. Although it is generally believed that pretesting is not helpful, Yocum and others (Yocum et al 1978) showed the value of a prolonged protocol of intravenous injections of serial dilutions of the contrast in predicting 'reactors' and also the value of antihistamine and corticosteroid premedication in preventing severe contrast media reactions. To be effective the corticosteroid should be given in full dosage for 3 days prior to the contrast. Metrizamide and more recently Iopamidol (Thomson & Schering 1987) have been shown to cause less reaction than ionic media in patients with a definite prior history of contrast medium reaction. Iopamidol is recommended for all patients in whom a contrast medium reaction may be expected.

The actual mechanism of 'contrast medium allergy' is uncertain and while some subscribe to the view that they are precipitated by patient apprehension (Lalli 1980) and prevented by intravenous diazepam, most believe that a complex reaction involving protein binding of the contrast and activation of bradykinin and other systems is responsible (Brash 1980). This latter view is supported by the onset of contrast reactions several hours after the contrast was given.

Treatment of contrast media reactions is discussed in Chapter 1.

POST-ANGIOGRAM CARE

After the angiogram is completed and haemostasis achieved the patient is kept in a supine position for 4 hours. It is our firm belief that the radiologist should compress the puncture site until the bleeding has stopped. This usually takes 10 minutes.

The puncture site, distal pulses, radial pulse and systemic blood pressure are examined and recorded every 5 minutes for 30 minutes then every 30 minutes for 30 hours. In the case of carotid angiography routine neurological observations are also made at the same intervals. Outpatients are assessed at this time and are usually allowed to go home at 4–6 hours after the examination is completed. (A maximum catheter size of 5F is used for outpatients.) Inpatients are kept in bed until 0800 hours the next day even if they were examined in the morning simply as a matter of nursing convenience. Patients who are unable to void may get out of bed to do so.

A bandage over the puncture is not used and if bleeding occurs then the artery is compressed by hand until the bleeding stops. A bandage tight enough to effectively compress the artery may cause occlusion of the distal vessels particularly if they are diseased and the distal flow is slow. In our view, none of the commercially available arterial compression devices is satisfactory.

Patients who have had axillary (brachial) punctures are not confined to bed but the arm is kept in a sling until the next morning at 0800 hours.

If only the femoral vein has been punctured the patient may ambulate after 30–60 minutes depending on the size of the catheterization.

Although a flexible post-angiogram protocol is convenient for the patient it may not be practical in a busy nursing situation and the actual care our patients receive is probably more uniform than stated above.

ANAESTHESIA AND ANALGESIA FOR ANGIOGRAPHY

For most patients the most painful part of the angiography is the flat hard examination table. The pain of the contrast injections is brief and usually well tolerated. Insertion of the catheter should not be a procedure which

requires general anaesthesia. Adequate analgesia can be provided for these
if required without rendering the patient unconscious (Spigos et al 1980).
    The indications for neurolept or general anaesthesia are:
1. An uncooperative patient or one who is likely to become so.
2. Very long procedures such as detachable balloon occlusion of carotico-
    cavernous fistulae.
3. Procedures in which severe pain will be produced as a result of the
    procedure. The most common examples are: (i) external carotid embo-
    lization for head and neck tumours and (ii) angiography of the hand.
    In some centres general anaesthesia is used routinely for all angiography.
In our view this lengthens the procedure and places the patient at risk of
anaesthetic as well as angiographic complications.
    A major objection to general anaesthesia, in our view, is the habit of
anaesthetists of turning the patient on their side with the hips flexed as soon
as the patient awakes. This position is not satisfactory to minimize the
chance of bleeding from the femoral puncture.
    Patients who have had a long neuroleptanaesthesia may develop very deep
sighing respirations which may make a delicate catheterization of an artery
to an abdominal viscus difficult or impossible. This also makes transhepatic
procedures dangerous.

SPECIFIC STUDIES

SINGLE LIMB ARTERIOGRAM

Lower limb with retrograde approach

Indications

Peripheral vascular disease prior to surgery or angioplasty. After trauma
where the circulation is impaired. To demonstrate the anatomy prior to
plastic reconstructive surgery. Occasionally in tumours or arteriovenous
malformations.

Patient preparation

Standard preparation. For a few minutes before the injection exercise the
patient's foot. This causes dilation of the small vessels and improves their
filling with contrast. Alternatively the leg may be made more ischaemic by
occluding the inflow with a pressure cuff for 5 minutes and producing
reactive hyperaemia. If this fails then a vasodilator may be used.

Technique

    1. Approach. Standard femoral retrograde approach.
    2. Catheter. A 5F polyethylene catheter 55 cm in length with 5 side
hole near the tip.

3. Wire guide. Teflon coated 'J-tip' with 1.5 mm curve radius 0.89 mm diameter and 145 cm long.

4. Site of injection. External iliac artery on the ipsilateral side.

5. Contrast. Iopamiro 300: 25 ml at 5 ml/second.

6. Exposure sequence

```
[TIME (seconds)]
0  1  2  3  4  5  6  7  8  9  10 11 12 13 14 15 16 17 18 19
[INJECTOR]
***********
[EXPOSURE]
   *    *    *    *              *                   *
: GROIN : THIGH : KNEE : TIBIA : ANKLE/FOOT :
[MOVEMENT]
          *         *         *         *
```

A second injection may be made with the patient in an oblique or lateral projection particularly for suspected femoral artery dissection or prior to plastic surgery. Generally these extra views are not necessary for the usual patient with peripheral disease.

Equipment

The most convenient method employs a programmed table and an automatic rate-controlled contrast injector, but this type of angiography can be performed less elegantly with multiple injections and repeated bucky exposures. In such cases lead shielding allows two exposures to be made per 35 × 42 cm film. In other centres long (90 cm) films or a cassette tunnel is used to increase the film available and limit the number of injections required.

Technical problems

Failure to opacify the arteries adequately is the most common problem. To avoid this a long bolus is used but if desired the transit can be timed with a test injection.

Unfortunately timing of a small test is not always the same as a larger injection. If the foot is severely ischaemic fluoroscopy of a test bolus may indicate the area of obstruction at which the filming should be concentrated. It is essential to keep track of the time at which the exposures were made and the rate at which the contrast was injected. This is much easier when the sequence is programmed.

Complications

If a needle is used for the injections of contrast the risk of extravasation is higher than when catheters are used, particularly if the patient is moved.

Puncture of prosthetic materials is more difficult but not contraindicated. A longer compression of the artery will be required for haemostasis. A false aneurysm is more likely if the artery is calcified or ectatic. A large groin haematoma makes any subsequent surgical dissection more awkward.

The examination which does not detail the disease accurately may be considered a complication. Particular care should be made to ensure that sections of the artery have not been missed due to insufficient overlap of films. This is more likely if the examination was performed without a programmed table or long film changer.

Lower limb with antegrade approach

Indications

1. Prior to lower limb angioplasty.
2. Popliteal aneurysms with poor run-off.
3. Intervention angiography (streptokinase, embolization).

Patient preparation

Standard.

Technique

1. Approach. Antegrade femoral.

2. Catheter. A 5F polyethylene catheter 55 cm in length with no side holes and a 1 cm diameter curve at the tip. This is shaped with boiling water at the time of use.

3. Wire guide. Teflon coated 'J-tip' with a 1.5 mm curve radius 0.89 mm diameter and 145 cm long. A Teflon coated 'long (10 cm) floppy tip' 0.89 mm diameter and 145 cm long if a distal position of the wire guide is required.

4. Site of injection. This varies with the clinical indications but generally as close to the site of disease as is possible.

5. Contrast. Iopamiro 300. The rate depends on the arterial flow. For an arteriovenous malformation a rapid injection (10 ml/s) is required but for a popliteal aneurysm a slow injection is indicated (5 ml/s).

6. Exposure sequence. In most cases the same program can be used for antegrade as retrograde lower limb angiograms. However a faster program should be used without movements in the case of an arteriovenous malformation and truncated program of one or two exposures is used for post-angioplasty angiography.

Equipment

The same as for 'Lower limb with retrograde approach' (see p. 77).

Technical problems

The most common problem is catheterization of the profunda femoris artery when the superficial femoral was equired. If the catheter is in the profunda femoris then it is withdrawn under fluoroscopy and the tip rotated until it is directed towards the superficial femoral artery. (This is one reason for the curve on the tip of the catheter.) The 'long floppy tip' wire guide and then the catheter are advanced down to the desired position. This technique requires puncture above the common femoral bifurcation. Turning the patient into the opposite posterior oblique will open the common femoral bifurcation and make this technique easier.

In the obese patient it may be difficult or impossible to perform an antegrade puncture because of their protruberant abdomen. In these patients it may be preferable to pass a catheter over the aortic bifurcation from the other side. In most patients the catheter needs to be 100 cm in length to reach the knee from the opposite femoral artery.

Complications

Dissection of the arterial wall is more serious with antegrade catheterizations because the flow of blood tends to open the dissection and cause occlusion of the artery.

Otherwise the complications are as for retrograde femoral catheterization.

AORTOGRAM AND BILATERAL FEMORAL ANGIOGRAM

Indications

These are the same as those for single limb angiography except that more information is required. In particular the status of the renal arteries and the lower aorta must be shown.

Patient preparation

The patient should not be dehydrated but solid food is not permitted for 4 hours prior to the examination. This is only to minimize the chance of aspiration should the patient vomit. Bowel preparation is not necessary.

Technique

Since most patients have impaired circulation a high injection rate is not required. An injection of contrast (Iopamiro 300: 30 ml) is made at 15 ml/s and one film exposed at the end of the injection. This is the effective maximum through a 5F catheter 55 cm long with 5 side holes at 600 psi.

The catheter is withdrawn to below the renal arteries but above the aortic bifurcation and a second injection of contrast (Iopamiro 300: 70 ml) made at 7 ml/s with the table programmed to move 3 to 4 times depending on the length of the patient.

1. Approach. The artery with the best pulse and without bruits is preferable. If the femoral pulses are poor or absent then an axillary or translumbar approach is indicated.

2. Catheter. A 5F polyethylene catheter 55 cm in length with 5 side holes near the tip.

3. Wire guide. Teflon coated 'J-tip' with 1.5 mm curve radius 0.89 mm diameter and 145 cm in length.

4. Site of injection. 1st injection: At the level of the renal arteries (see Fig. 4.8).
2nd injection: Midway between the renal arteries and the aortic bifurcation. With translumbar and axillary punctures the contrast is injected above or at the level of the renal arteries.

5. Contrast. 1st injection: 30 ml Iopamiro 300 at 15 ml/s.
2nd injection: 70 ml Iopamiro 300 at 7 ml/s.

6. Exposure sequence. 1st injection: A single exposure at the end of the injection. (2 s.)
2nd injection: A series for the femoral arteries.

```
[TIME (seconds)]
0  1  2  3  4  5  6  7  8  9  10 11 12 13 14 15 16 17 18 19
[INJECTOR]
***********************
[EXPOSURE]
        *    *         *         *         *
: PELVIS : THIGH : KNEE : TIBIA : ANKLE :
[TABLE MOVEMENT]
        *    *    *         *
```

Sometimes the common femoral bifurcation will not be shown in an AP projection and a further injection of contrast in the appropriate posterior oblique is required. The film run may either extend down the leg or be truncated to cover only the area required. In truncated programs the injection of contrast may be smaller in volume and higher in rate of delivery (40 ml at 20 ml/s).

```
[TIME (seconds)]
0  1  2  3  4  5  6  7  8  9  10 11 12 13 14 15 16 17 18 19
[INJECTOR]
***********************
[EXPOSURE]
        *   *   *   *         *     *           *
*
         : ABDOMEN : PELVIS : THIGH : KNEES & TIBIAE : ANKLE :
           *                 *        *              *
```

The translumbar/axillary program is also used with femoral catheterizations

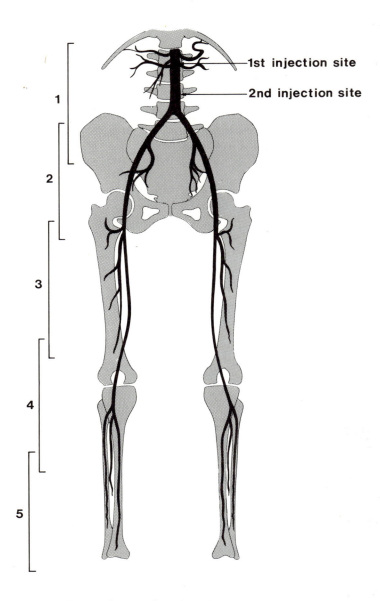

Fig. 4.8 *Schematic diagram of an aortofemoral arteriogram.*
 The first injection site is for a high rate injection to show the renal arteries. The second injection site is for a low rate injection to produce adequate opacification of the distal vessels. The numbers on the left margin refer to the film sequence and the position of exposures.

when the blood flow appears slow clinically or if there are advanced
ischaemic changes in the legs.

Equipment

This technique requires a programed table and automatic rate-controlled
injector with a capacity of at least 100 ml. It can be performed if the patient
is manually moved between exposures (see Fig. 4.9) but the injector is
essential. Most gas-powered injectors have a 50 ml capacity and are not
suitable for this long slow injection method.

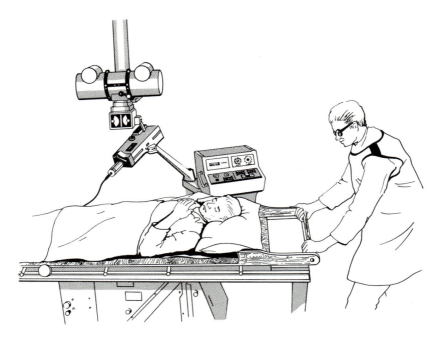

Fig. 4.9 *Technician powered moveable table top.*
    During the injection of contrast the X-ray technician moves the patient by moving a
plywood tray supported on dowelling rollers. Adequate radiation protection for the
technician is essential.

Technical problems

Timing of exposures is not a great problem if the long slow injection technique is used. If there is great disparity between the flow in each leg then
two separate injections and film runs may be required.
    In some patients the iliac arteries are so tortuous that catheterization is
difficult or impossible. If one side is impassable the other side is worth

trying before proceeding to axillary or translumbar puncture (Hessel & Sequira 1981). The catheter should be inserted on the side of the strongest pulse and the presence of an iliac bruit is an indication to use the other side. A single end hole 5F catheter with a curved tip is advanced to the first bend or obstruction and contrast injected to demonstrate the problem. Rotation of the catheter will direct the wire guide past the lesion. A 'J-tip' wire guide is used for tortuosity and a 'long floppy tip' wire guide for stenosis. In extreme cases the catheter may be advanced gently under fluoroscopy while contrast is continuously injected. If a very narrow stenosis is passed, an injection of contrast should be made to ensure that the blood flow to the leg is not occluded. Once the aorta is reached the end hole catheter is exchanged for the 5 side hole catheter and the examination completed. If one side proves impassable then the opposite side is worth trying without delay (Lalli 1980).

Complications

Most complications are related to sub-intimal dissection in the iliac arteries or dislodgement of atheroma from the lower aorta. Rarely a massive embolization of the lower limbs may occur with small atheromatous emboli from presumably the lower aorta.

Contrast staining of the aortic wall may occur but is not usually associated with morbidity.

Acute renal failure has been recorded after aortography and appears to be related to patient hydration and contrast dose to the kidneys. The exact mechanism is unclear but it may be a direct toxic effect of the contrast (Ansari & Baldwin 1976, Older et al 1980).

Translumbar puncture is always associated with a local haematoma of moderate size and damage to the origins of aortic branches may occur. A large sub-intimal injection could occlude the aorta but in practice this should be avoided by the performance of a test injection.

Complications particular to trans-axillary puncture include stroke and damage to the brachial plexus or the median nerve in addition to local arterial damage at the puncture site.

AORTOGRAM — ABDOMINAL

Indications

Patients with suspected stenosis or occlusion of the renal coeliac or mesenteric arteries and in cases of abdominal trauma.

Prior to more selective angiography if the anatomy is atypical or if the clinical localization is limited. With computerized tomography this is less an indication than in the past particularly in respect to renal and adrenal tumours.

In type III aortic dissection to delineate the inferior extent. (The catheter should be left proximal to the dissection so that both channels are filled with contrast.)

Patient preparation

Standard.

Technique

1. Approach. Retrograde femoral or axillary as indicated by the state of the iliac arteries or any subsequent selective catheterization. It is easier to catheterize some arteries from above.

2. Catheter. A 6.5F polyethylene catheter 55 cm in length with 5 side holes near the tip. Alternatively 'highflow' 4 or 5F polyurethane catheters may be used in the same configuration.

3. Wire guide. Teflon coated 'J-tip' with 1.5 mm curve radius 0.89 mm diameter and 145 cm in length.

4. Site of injection. Above the coeliac artery usually at the lower border of the 11th thoracic vertebral body.

5. Contrast. Iopamiro 370. 50–60 ml at 25–30 ml/s depending on the size of the patient.

6. Exposure sequence. View a satisfactory 'scout' film prior to the injection of contrast to avoid unnecessary repeats.

```
[TIME (seconds)]
0  1  2  3  4  5  6  7  8  9  10 11 12 13 14 15 16 17 18 19
[INJECTOR]
★★★★★
[EXPOSURE]
★★★   ★     ★    ★
(3/s)
```

In some cases an oblique or lateral projection is indicated especially if coeliac or mesenteric artery origin stenosis is suspected. If severe occlusive disease is found a 'customized' exposure sequence should be created and the injection of contrast repeated.

Equipment

A rapid film changing system of at least 3/s is essential. The examination is usually recorded on 35 cm × 35 cm film but 70–100 mm film cameras have been used. The major objection to film cameras in most cases is the limited field of view.

Technical problems

An aortogram is usually a simple procedure. If a general survey film is required avoid excessive limitation of the field size as a vital area may be excluded unintentionally. The gonads should be shielded as this examination is often performed on young adults.

Complications

There is none exclusive to abdominal aortography.

AORTOGRAM — THORACIC

Indications

Suspected aortic dissection in which case the examination must include the ascending aorta (and the abdominal aorta if dissection is found).

Aneurysms and coarctation of the aorta

Investigation of thoracic arteriovenous malformation and as a survey prior to bronchial arteriography in selected cases.

Patient preparation

Standard preparation.

Technique

It is essential that at least two projections at right angles are obtained especially if an aortic dissection is suspected clinically. If the chest roentgenogram shows an abnormal shadow in a particular projection it is useful to perform the angiogram in that projection also. (Usually AP.)

Assessment of aortic incompetence is part of a thoracic aortogram and the catheter should be positioned with this in mind.

1. Approach. Retrograde femoral approach. In coarctation a brachial or right axillary may be indicated on clinical grounds.

2. Catheter. The catheter used should be capable of a flow rate of 25 ml/s. An 8F polyethylene catheter 100 cm in length with 5 side holes near the tip in straight or 'pigtail' configuration are generally used. Polyurethane 'highflow' catheters of 5 or 6.5F size may be used instead. The connectors used must be capable of withstanding the pressures generated by the injector (800–1000 psi).

3. Wire guide. Teflon coated 'J-tip' with 1.5 mm curve radius 0.89 mm diameter and 145 cm in length. In young patients a 'wide (15 mm radius) J-tip' wire guide may be required to gain access to the ascending aorta as a straight wire guide will engage the left subclavian artery and often the vertebral artery also.

4. *Site of injection.* Ascending aorta close to the aortic valve or in the proximal descending aorta depending on the clinical indications.

5. *Contrast.* Iopamiro 370. (50–60 ml at 24–30 ml/s.)

6. *Exposure sequence*

[TIME (seconds)]
0 1 2 3 4 5 6 7 8 9 10 11 12 13 14 15 16 17 18 19
[INJECTOR]
****
[EXPOSURE]
****** * * *

Equipment

A rapid film changer and automatic rate-controlled injector are required.

Technical problems

In young patients with high cardiac outputs the contrast may be intermittently diluted with ventricular systole. This problem is minimized with injection rates of 30 ml/s. If a straight catheter is used care should be exercised to ensure that the tip is not in a position to deliver a large bolus of contrast directly into one of the coronary arteries.

Complications

In addition to those associated with abdominal aortography there is a risk of cerebral complications since the catheter is positioned 'upstream' of the carotid and vertebral arteries. Catheter aspiration and flushing with separate syringes as for carotid angiography should be performed.

If the catheter crosses the aortic valve it may cause ventricular arrhythmia until it is withdrawn. Positioning a catheter in the left ventricular cavity should only be performed intentionally with ECG monitoring and a defibrillator nearby.

AORTOGRAM — AORTIC ARCH STUDIES

Indications

Stenosis or occlusion of the branches of the aortic arch.

Patient preparation

Standard preparation.

Technique

As for thoracic aortography. See preceding section.

This examination may be performed alone or in combination with selective carotid angiography. Usually both right and left posterior oblique projections are performed.

The examination should extend from the arch vessel origins to the carotid bifurcations and the distal subclavian arteries bilaterally.

Image quality is improved if the X-ray beam is smoothed by adding density to the neck area by aluminium wedges on the X-ray tube face or flourbags on the patient. Subtraction films are usually required particularly for the carotid bifurcation. The patient should be instructed to suspend respiration and swallowing during filming.

Equipment

Same as for thoracic aortogram.

Technical problems

Patient motion may prevent good subtraction and the wide variation in density of the area being examined makes an evenly exposed roentgenogram difficult to obtain. The carotid and vertebral origins are often not shown to advantage and at least two views are required in almost all cases. The dose of contrast required is high and it is not always possible to repeat injections if the patient is in incipient heart failure.

Complications

Same as for thoracic aortogram.

SELECTIVE ABDOMINAL ANGIOGRAPHY

Selective angiography involves the placement of a catheter usually with a single end hole into a branch of the aorta or into a subdivision of the branch itself. This is the most difficult part of angiography from a technical point of view.

The degree of difficulty depends on the tortuosity of the vessels to be catheterized, the size of the target artery and the distance from the aorta. A single curve is usually easy to negotiate but an 'S-bend' is not.

General technique

In most cases the easiest approach is from the femoral route, but if the artery has a steep downward angle of origin from the aorta then an approach from the axillary artery may be indicated. If multiple catheter changes are to be made then an arterial sheath set with a flushing side arm should be considered to minimize trauma to the artery. The sheath set also reduces the likelihood of arterial spasm at the puncture site. The major disadvantage is the sheath is at least one French size bigger than the catheter which can be inserted through it.

When a sheath is used or when the selective catheterization is expected to take longer than 30 minutes, consideration should be given to anti-coagulation of the patient with 5000 IU of heparin given intravenously. In very long cases an infusion of 1000 IU hourly should be given after the initial dose. At the end of the procedure the heparin can be reversed with protamine 1 mg/1000 IU of active heparin. Protamine should be given very slowly intravenously. No protamine is required if the heparin was last given more than 45 minutes previously.

Specific techniques

Antegrade

A curved catheter is positioned at the orifice of the artery and a 'long floppy' wire guide 0.89 mm diameter is advanced into the artery. The catheter is then advanced over the wire guide into the artery. The tip of the wire guide should be maintained in position by withdrawing it slightly as the catheter is advanced. Often a gentle reciprocating motion of the catheter on the wire guide will aid advancement.

Retrograde

A catheter with a long recurved tip is used to engage the artery from the aorta above its origin and the catheter is withdrawn to advance the tip into the artery. Generally the length of the recurved portion limits the amount of selectivity. Insertion of a wire guide usually straightens the catheter tip unless a moveable core wire guide is used.

Coaxial

This method uses a large (6–7F) outer catheter which is placed in the artery using an antegrade technique and a smaller inner catheter which is advanced using a selection of torque wire guides (Cope–Eisenberg System: Elecath Inc.). The system uses a series of Tuohy–Borst adapters to allow flushing of the inner and outer catheters.

Fig. 4.10 (right) *Catheterization of the coeliac artery with a looped cobra catheter.*
Panel 1. The catheter is inserted well into the superior mesenteric artery. *Panel 2.* Continued advancement cause the catheter to form a loop up the aorta. *Panel 3.* The catheter is advanced further so that the tip lies above the coeliac artery orifice. *Panel 4.* As the catheter is withdrawn the tip engages the coeliac artery and moves down it. Insertion of more catheter at the groin puncture will disengage the catheter from the coeliac artery.

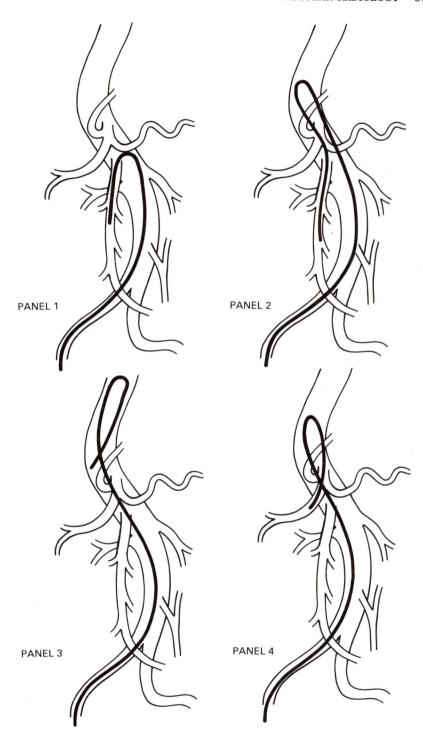

PANEL 1

PANEL 2

PANEL 3

PANEL 4

Other

Any or all of these techniques may be used in a difficult catheterization. A braided polyethylene 6.5F catheter (Cook BPS 'Torcon') can be used for an antegrade technique, curved in the renal or superior mesenteric arteries to produce a recurved catheter for a retrograde technique and if necessary a 3F catheter may be passed through the 6.5F catheter for a coaxial technique. This is the method we prefer in the first instance.

To produce a recurved catheter a 'loop' technique is performed as follows: a braided polyethylene (Cook BPS) 6.5F 'Cobra' catheter 80 cm in length with a single end hole is inserted into the superior mesenteric or other suitable artery (renal, splenic, or contralateral common iliac artery) and the 'long floppy' wire guide advanced for several centimetres beyond the catheter into the artery (see Fig. 4.10). By advancing the catheter a long recurved loop is produced in the catheter. The length of the loop should be at least 10 cm as a shorter loop will curl on itself in the aorta. Rotating the catheter 180° and advancing it further will cause it to disengage and lie free in the aorta. The catheter, with the wire guide still in place but withdrawn into the catheter tip, is directed towards the target artery orifice from above and withdrawn to engage the catheter in the artery. If necessary the wire guide may be advanced slightly from the catheter to facilitate this procedure. If the wire guide is removed completely, when it is replaced, it may straighten the loop.

A very wide range of catheters in various shapes and wire guides of many types are available for use in selective angiography. In any particular instance several of these may be tried. If a catheter and wire guide combination does not work fairly quickly it is better to use either a different catheter or wire guide rather than to persist for a very long time with the same catheter.

RENAL ARTERIOGRAPHY

Standard method

Indications

The indications for renal arteriography have been modified by the use of computed tomography and ultrasound and simple renal or adrenal tumours no longer require arteriography prior to surgery if an adequate CT scan has been performed.
1. Suspected renal artery stenosis prior to angioplasty.
2. Renal parenchymal disease (including renal tumours).
3. Gross unexplained haematuria. (In combination with renal venography.)
4. Severe renal trauma.
5. Prior to renal artery embolization for haematuria or tumour.

Patient preparation

Standard preparation. If a phaeochromotoma is suspected clinically the patient should receive an alpha and beta adrenergic blockade given by a separate physician to the radiologist and an intravenous line should be open. An abdominal CT scan should be performed prior to selective studies in such cases as the tumours are often large and very vascular and angiography is often not required.

Technique

1. *Approach.* In most cases the renal arteries can be catheterized easily from the femoral artery by withdrawing the catheter from above the level of the renal arteries while directing the tip laterally. In most cases a preliminary aortogram is not required as the position of the renal arteries is fairly constant.

2. *Catheter.* Braided polyethylene (Cook BPS) 6.5F 'Cobra' 80 cm in length with a single end hole.

3. *Wire guide.* Teflon coated 'J-tip' with a 1.5 mm curve radius 0.89 mm diameter, and a Teflon coated straight 'long floppy' wire guide 0.89 mm diameter, both 145 cm in length. The 'J-tip' is used for the aortic catheterization and the 'long floppy' wire guide is used only if necessary for the selective catheterization of the renal artery.

4. *Site of injection.* Main renal artery or more peripherally as indicated.

5. *Contrast.* Urografin 76 (10 ml at 6–8 ml/s) for most cases. A smaller slower injection is used for sub-selective injections.

6. *Exposure sequence*

[TIME (seconds)]
0 1 2 3 4 5 6 7 8 9 10 11 12 13 14 15 16 17 18 19
[INJECTOR]
★★★★
[EXPOSURE]
★★★★   ★   ★
(3/s)

Equipment

A rapid film changer is most suitable. The contrast may be injected by hand but this subjects the operator to unnecessary radiation exposure. Magnification angiography should be performed in all cases of parenchymal disease and in cases of haematuria.

When the angle of origin of the renal artery is acute, the catheter can be inserted into the renal artery from above either using a 'loop' technique or from the axillary artery.

Except in cases of renal tumour, when the renal vein and inferior vena cava should be included, the X-ray beam should be coned to the renal area. The adrenal glands should always be included.

Catheter recoil during injection is avoided by inserting the catheter further but not beyond an early origin of a branch of the renal artery. In patients with fibromuscular dysplasia the examination should be performed in deep inspiration to 'stretch' the renal artery.

Usually an AP and an oblique view are required. The oblique should display the sinus of the kidney in profile and the degree of angulation is best determined under fluoroscopy following test injections of contrast.

Multiple renal arteries are common. If the branches are small a hand injection of contrast and a film camera may be used. The selective angiographic appearance of multiple renal arteries is characteristic.

Complications

Acute renal failure may follow any abdominal angiography and the dose of contrast delivered to the kidney should be kept to a practical minimum.

Injection of contrast through 'wedged' catheters may cause rupture of the artery. Intimal dissection of the renal artery is usually the result of vigorous wire guide manipulation. Concentrated heparin should not be injected directed into the renal or any other artery.

Other techniques

Procedures

These are usually preceded by standard selective renal arteriography.
1. High volume injections of contrast to show the renal vein in renal tumours. (Without adrenaline.)
2. Adrenaline enhanced angiography of hypovascular renal tumours.

Patient preparation

Adrenaline should be given with care in patients with heart disease.

Standard preparation. The patient should be warned that they may experience a feeling of acute anxiety following the adrenaline injection.

Other vasoconstrictors such as angiotensin II may be used instead.

Technique

1. Approach. As for 'Standard method' above (see p. 62). If it is indicated, adrenaline 5–10 μg is given through the selective catheter 20–30 seconds before the injection of contrast. To provide a convenient adrenaline injection mix 0.5 ml of 1:1000 adrenaline in a bottle of 500 ml of normal saline. The resulting mixture contains 1 μg of adrenaline per ml.

2. Contrast. Large volume to show the renal vein: Urografin 76 20–5 ml at 8–10 ml/s. Adrenaline enhanced: Urografin 76 5–10 ml at 2–4 ml/s.

3. Exposure sequence

[TIME (seconds)]
0 1 2 3 4 5 6 7 8 9 10 11 12 13 14 15 16 17 18 19
[INJECTOR]
****
[EXPOSURE]
  ★ ★ ★ ★   ★   ★   ★   ★

Technical problems

Very large tumours may be too large for a magnification series. Generally a non-magnified film is adequate in large tumours.

Intro-arterial adrenaline decreases the rate of flow through the kidney and a rapid injection will outline the aorta instead of the kidney. Since the vessels being sought are small, magnification films are essential.

A delay of about 15 minutes is preferable between injections of adrenaline and the pulse and blood pressure should be monitored. No more than two injections should be necessary.

Complications

A large dose of contrast in a renal tumour which is soon to be removed is not likely to cause problems. If the patient has been given adrenaline in excessive amounts there will be signs of increased sympathomimetic activity. These are a cold clammy skin with a rapid pulse and an elevated blood pressure. If the patient develops angina a sublingual nitroglycerine tablet is given.

COELIAC ARTERIOGRAPHY

Indications

1. Bleeding from the upper gastrointestinal tract.
2. Arterial anatomy of hepatic, pancreatic and splenic masses.
3. Demonstration of the portal vein in portal hypertension.
4. Severe blunt abdominal trauma.
5. Prior to hepatic infusion of cytotoxic drugs.

Patient preparation

Standard

The stomach and duodenum may be distended with gas and paralyzed with

Buscopan or Glucagon during angiography of pancreatic tumours or in some cases of slow gastro-duodenal haemorrhage.

Technique

1. Approach. Generally standard femoral approach but a 'loop' technique is usually required if the patient is over 50 years or if the liver or spleen are enlarged. In a young adult the catheter is inserted into the aorta and the tip placed above the twelfth thoracic vertebral body. The catheter tip is rotated anteriorly and gently withdrawn. As the catheter flicks into the coeliac orifice the motion can be seen fluoroscopically and felt with the finders. A small contrast injection will confirm the catheter position.

2. Catheter. Braided polyethylene (Cook BPS) 6.5F 'Cobra' catheter 80 cm in length with a single end hole. A short (No. 1) curve is used in a narrow aorta.

Preshaped recurved catheters in braided polyethylene 'Sidewinder Type' are also useful but they will usually not engage further than the length of the preshaped tip without effort.

A 'Cope-Eisenberg' co-axial system is required for pancreatic arteriography.

3. Wire guide. Teflon coated 'J-tip' with 1.5 mm curve radius 0.89 mm diameter for the aortic catheterization, and a Teflon coated straight 'long floppy' wire guide 0.89 mm diameter for the selective catheterization. Occasionally a 'moveable core' straight wire guide is used for super-selective catheterization and 'deflector tip' wire guide is used to insert the catheter into the coeliac orifice.

4. Site of injection. In cases of bleeding the initial injection should fill the left gastric artery which arises close to the origin of the coeliac artery itself. For best demonstration of the portal vein the injection should be as close to the spleen as possible. Since the left gastric artery may supply the liver in cases of hepatic tumour the injection should include the common hepatic and left gastric arteries.

5. Contrast. Iopamiro 370.
Coeliac trunk: 35 ml at 10 ml/s
Common hepatic artery: 35 ml at 10 ml/s
Splenic artery: 45 ml at 10–12 ml/s
Other arteries: variable depending on size
The injector should be connected directly to the catheter for rates in excess of 10 ml/s.

6. Exposure sequence

[TIME (seconds)]
0 1 2 3 4 5 6 7 8 9 10 11 12 13 14 15 16 17 18 19
[INJECTOR]
****
[EXPOSURE]
  * * *   *   *   *   *   *   *

Equipment

Rapid film changer and automatic rate controlled injector. This and most other exposure sequences are designed to allow two film runs with subtraction films per film magazine (Puck or AOT Film changers).

Technical problems

There is a very high incidence of anatomical variations in the coeliac axis of which the most common is origin of the hepatic artery from the superior mesenteric artery. The angiographer should be familiar with these (Michels 1955).

The coeliac artery arises a little to the left of the midline normally and much more if the liver is enlarged. Splenic enlargement causes a sharp curve in the coeliac artery – splenic artery junction. In such cases a 'loop' catheter technique is required. In extreme cases the axillary approach is necessary.

Selective catheterization of the left gastric artery is performed by either straightening the curve at the tip of the catheter with the stiff end of the wire guide or by reforming a loop catheter in the hepatic artery and engaging the left gastric as the catheter is 'advanced' out of the coeliac axis (see Fig. 4.11). Catheter recoil is common if the injection is made at the coeliac origin at a high rate unless the catheter has a 'shepherds crook' shape or a loop in the aorta to stabilize the tip.

Pancreatic arteriography may require extensive super-selective catheterization but it is rarely indicated since the advent of computed tomography.

When using a 'loop technique' a 'moveable core' wire guide may be used to lead the catheter tip without displacing the catheter. It is usually impossible to advance the mandrel once it has been withdrawn due to the curve of the catheter and artery.

Vasoconstrictor drugs may be used to enhance the demonstration of hypovascular tumours in the liver and a dose of 8–10 μg of adrenaline is given through the catheter 20 to 30 s before the injection of contrast (see 'Renal arteriography', p. 90). Vasopressin may be used for 'non-selective' pancreatic angiography as the pancreatic vessels contract less in response to vasopressin than do the splenic, hepatic and gastro-duodenal vessels.

Failure to show a bleeding vessel is most often due to the fact that the patient is no longer bleeding at the time of the arteriogram. It is not worth proceeding if the patient has no clinical evidence of active blood loss at the time. A radio-isotope scan is likely to be more useful than arteriography in very low rate bleeders. Slow bleeding may require very selective angiography.

Complications

Minor subintimal dissection is common during difficult catheterization of the coeliac axis but any effects are usually sub-clinical.

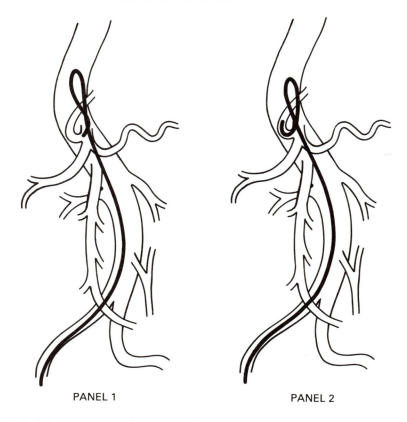

PANEL 1   PANEL 2

Fig. 4.11 *Left gastric artery catheterization with a looped cobra catheter.*
Panel 1. Beginning with a looped catheter further down the coeliac axis (see Fig. 4.10).
Insert more catheter at the groin to begin disengagement. As the catheter reaches the left
gastric artery orifice rotate the catheter slightly in the clockwise direction. *Panel 2.* Traction
on the catheter will cause it to move further into the left gastric artery. This is a very
stable catheter position.

Pancreatitis may occur after selective injections into the small pancreatic
arteries.

We have seen a catheter recoil violently from the coeliac axis during
contrast injection and the jet of contrast, or the catheter itself, dislodge
significant amounts of atheroma which then caused massive small vessel
embolization of the kidneys, bowel, and lower limbs. This is, however, very
unusual.

Time passes rapidly during a difficult catheterization and the use of
systemic heparin will minimize thrombotic complications during long
procedures.

SUPERIOR MESENTERIC ARTERIOGRAPHY

Indications

1. Bleeding from the upper gastrointestinal tract.
2. Vascular disorders of the upper gastrointestinal tract.
3. Demonstration of the portal venous system (in conjunction with the splenic arteriogram).
4. Severe blunt abdominal trauma.

Patient preparation

Standard preparation. In cases of haemorrhage the bowel may be paralysed with Buscopan or glucagon to improve detection of small lesions. A vasodilator is very useful in cases of ischaemia or when the portal system is being examined. The most convenient is tolazoline 10–25 mg as a bolus through the catheter about 30 s prior to the injection of contrast.

Technique

1. Approach. Standard femoral approach. The orifice of the superior mesenteric artery is usually found in the mid-line at the level of the first lumbar vertebra above the renal arteries.

2. Catheter. Braided polyethylene (Cook BPS) 6.5F 'Cobra' catheter 80 cm in length with a single end hole. Except in very small aortae the No. 2 shape is used.

3. Wire guide. Teflon coated 'J-tip' with 1.5 mm curve radius 0.89 mm diameter for the aortic catheterization, and a Teflon coated straight 'long floppy' wire guide 0.89 mm diameter for more selective catheterization.

4. Site of injection. Close to the origin of the vessel in the first instance unless a more distal site is indicated.

5. Contrast. Iopamiro 370. For most injections 35–45 ml at 10–12 ml/s unless a vasodilator has been given when the volume and rate may be increased.

6. Exposure sequence. This is the same as for the coeliac axis. See above.

Technical problems

The superior mesenteric artery is usually readily catheterized from below or above. When a 'loop' catheter is required to engage the superior mesenteric artery the look may be formed gently in a renal artery, across the aortic bifurcation, or with the help of a 'deflecting tip' wire guide. Deflecting-tip wire guides should be used in a wide portion of the aorta, if necessary in the thoracic aortic arch.

When the hepatic artery arises from the superior mesenteric artery it can be selectively catheterized by making a 'loop' in the superior mesenteric artery and withdrawing the tip from the superior mesenteric artery by advancing the catheter up the aorta. Once the catheter tip engages the hepatic artery withdrawing the catheter from the aorta will advance the tip into the hepatic artery.

Spasm may occur in the jejunal branches as a result of catheterization and sometimes will respond to intra-arterial nitroglycerine 50–100 μg in a bolus.

Complications

This examination is usually performed in concert with a coeliac arteriogram and the complications are common to both procedures.

INFERIOR MESENTERIC ARTERIOGRAPHY

Indications

1. Lower gastrointestinal bleeding or ischaemia.
2. Assessment of malignancy in colonic masses (rarely used).

Patient preparation

Standard preparation.

Technique

1. Approach. Standard femoral approach. Sometimes the examination may be easier from the left side particularly if the aorta is tortuous.

2. Catheter. Braided polyethylene (Cook BPS) 6.5F 'Rosch Inferior Mesenteric' (RIM) catheter 80 cm in length with a single end hole.

3. Wire guide. Teflon coated 'J-tip' with a 1.5 mm curve radius 0.89 mm diameter for aortic catheterization. A wire guide is not usually required to engage the inferior mesenteric artery with the catheter.

4. Site of injection. Proximal inferior mesenteric artery.

5. Contrast. Iopamiro 370. Volume of 15–20 ml delivered at 3–5 ml/s depending on the size of the artery.

6. Exposure sequence. Same as for coeliac and superior mesenteric arteriography.

Equipment

Same as for coeliac and superior mesenteric arteriography.

Technical problems

In patients with aortic aneurysms the inferior mesenteric artery may be occluded and even when it is not, it is difficult to see on abdominal aortography if it is small. Lateral fluoroscopy or rotating the patient 45° to their left will in most cases allow the artery to be seen following a test injection of contrast at the lower border of the second lumbar vertebra. Almost all inferior mesenteric arteries arise between the L2–L3 and L3–L4 disc spaces. The RIM catheter is designed to hook into the orifice in a stable position but it is not suited to super-selective catheterization. The torque control provided by the BPS catheter material has greatly simplified this examination.

The length of the left colic branch usually requires at least two injections of contrast because of the area to be examined. The left colon is examined in AP projection and the recto-sigmoid portion is examined in a steep left posterior oblique projection to 'open out' the sigmoid loop.

The recto-sigmoid portion should be examined first as the contrast filled bladder will overlay this region. If the coeliac and superior mesenteric arteries have already been examined the patient should attempt to void or the bladder drained by catheter before the inferior mesenteric artery is injected with contrast. The contrast injection will give the patient a feeling of rectal evacuation and they should be reassured before the injection that the sensation is not accompanied by the act.

Complications

Same as for coeliac and superior mesenteric arteriography.

SELECTIVE PELVIC ARTERIOGRAPHY

Indications

1. Bleeding after pelvic trauma.
2. Tumours of the uterus, ovaries or pelvic wall.
3. Ultrasound has replaced arteriorgraphy in the study of the pregnant uterus.

Patient preparation

Standard preparation.

Technique

1. Approach. Either femoral approach. A 'loop catheter technique' is used and the internal iliac arteries catheterized from above. The loop is reformed in the first side examined to enable the other side to be catheterized in the same fashion.

2. Catheter. Braided polyethylene (Cook BPS) 6.5F 'Cobra' 80 cm in length with a single end hole. Usually a No. 2 curve tip is used.

3. Wire guide. Teflon coated 'J-tip' with 1.5 mm curve radius 0.89 mm diameter for the aortic catheterization, and a Teflon coated straight 'long floppy' wire guide 0.89 mm diameter for the selective catheterization.

4. Site of injection. As indicated clinically.

5. Contrast. Iopamiro 370. The volume and rate vary considerably depending on the catheter position. For the internal iliac artery 25 ml at 10 ml/s may be used. An indication of the volume required may be obtained from test injections with fluoroscopy.

6. Exposure sequence

[TIME (seconds)]
0 1 2 3 4 5 6 7 8 9 10 11 12 13 14 15 16 17 18 19
[INJECTOR]
****
[EXPOSURE]
★ ★ ★ ★   ★   ★   ★   ★

Equipment

Rapid film changer and an automatic rate-controlled injector. In cases of tumour a subtraction film is useful.

Technical problems

The major difficulty is selecting the desired branch of the internal iliac artery. For this reason a film run at the start of the procedure is helpful to demonstrate the anatomy. For embolization of bleeding a super-selective technique is not required. The 6.5F catheter may wedge in very small vessels but in an adult, arteries the size of the uterine and obturator arteries may be catheterized without problems.

Complications

There are not any which are particular to selective pelvic arteriography.

CORONARY ARTERIOGRAPHY

Coronary arteriography is generally performed by cardiologists rather than by radiologists and this section is not intended to be comprehensive. Judkins' technique only will be described (Judkins 1967).

Indications

1. Investigation of chest pain in general and angina pectoris in particular.
2. Prior to cardiac valve surgery in adults.
3. After a sub-endocardial myocardial infarct.

Patient preparation

Standard preparation. Premedication of diazepam or an opiate with atropine is usual. A scalp vein needle is placed in a vein on the back of one hand for administration of drugs if necessary during the procedure.

The patient is anticoagulated with 5000 IU heparin intra-arterially at the beginning of the procedure and the anticoagulation reversed with protamine 20–40 mg at the conclusion. The protamine is given slowly intravenously.

Technique

1. Approach. Femoral approach or left axillary approach if Judkins' technique is used. Alternatively a brachial artery cutdown and Sone's technique may be used.

2. Catheter. Three catheters 120 cm in length are required. Generally much more rigid catheters are used for coronary angiography than for other angiography. Polyethylene catheters may be used for the left coronary artery and the left ventricle and a braided polyethylene catheter used for the right coronary artery. Some prefer to use three braided catheters but this significantly increases the catheter cost. A 7F size is sufficient for most cases except patients with aortic stenosis and very large coronary arteries. The Judkins catheter contains a secondary curve 3 to 6 cm long and the catheters are coded by the length of this curve. A 4 cm curve suits most people but a 5 cm curve may be required if the aorta is dilated. A pigtail catheter with 5 side holes is used for the left ventricular and aortic injections. A 7F coronary artery 'set' is available (Cook Australia).

3. Wire guide. Teflon coated 'J-tip' with 1.5 mm curve radius, 145 cm long and 0.89 mm diameter.

4. Site of injection. Hand injections are made in several projections through the coronary catheters engaged in the orifice of each coronary artery. The left ventricular injection is made with an injector.

5. Contrast. Iopamiro 370. If an ionic contrast is used instead then the ratio of sodium to methylgulcamine ions in the contrast medium is important and not all contrast media are suitable. This is discussed in the chapter on contrast media.

6. Exposure sequence. Almost all examinations are made with cinefluoroscopy rather than rapid film changers. The film should be running before the injection starts and after the injection ends. An average case will use 70–90 m of 35 mm film exposed at 50 frames/s.

Equipment

Continuous electrocardiographic and catheter-tip pressure monitoring is essential as the catheter is not flushed at intervals and generally left in the coronary orifice or left ventricle until that part of the examination is completed. If the ECG changes or the pressure drops the catheter is withdrawn. A technician is usually committed to observing the monitors throughout the procedure.

Technical problems

Unless thwarted by the operator the left Judkins catheter will engage the left coronary orifice simply by being advanced up the aorta. Care should be exercised to ensure that the catheter does not wedge or dissect the coronary orifice. If the catheter goes past the orifice it usually engages it as the catheter is withdrawn slowly. In the left anterior projection the catheter can be adjusted easily to ensure that it has not been rotated inadvertently.

The right Judkins catheter must be rotated 180° about 8–10 cm above the right coronary orifice and as it rotates it will descend without further advancement from the groin. Over-rotation and over-insertion before rotation are the major causes of difficulty. Catheterization of the right coronary artery is easier in the left anterior oblique projection as this profiles the proximal portion of the artery.

The pigtail catheter may cause ventricular tachycardia or extrasystoles when in the ventricle and it should be withdrawn or rotated into a position which does not irritate the ventricle. The area below the mitral valve is often satisfactory.

Complications

Several times each year bubbles of air are injected into coronary arteries without ill effect but they may cause serious ischaemia and they should be avoided if possible. Blood product emboli are usually the cause of myocardial infarction but are rare due to the routine use of anticoagulation.

Arrhythmias (and in particular ventricular fibrillation) may follow cardiac catheterization and coronary injections of contrast. When the arrhythmia has been treated successfully (if necessary by DC defibrillation) the examination can continue. Ventricular fibrillation appears to be much less common than it once was.

Hypotension may place the patient with severe coronary disease in a position in which there is severe coronary insufficiency. As it is usual to give the patient sub-lingual nitroglycerine during the examination aliquots of aramine 0.5–1.0 mg may be given to maintain the blood pressure at pre-nitroglycerine levels.

In patients with left main coronary disease great care should be exercised to ensure that the catheter is not wedged and the absolute minimum number of injections of contrast made. We recommend shallow right anterior oblique, cranially angulated left anterior oblique and lateral projections. If the stenosis is severe the opacification of the distal vessels may be less than usual but this is not improved by more or longer injections which may be hazardous for the patient.

The complications of thoracic arch aortography also apply.

MISCELLANEOUS SELECTIVE ANGIOGRAPHY

In this section only the variation from standard procedures is specified.

Bronchial arteriography

Indications

1. Persistent haemoptysis (in cystic fibrosis).
2. Diagnosis and cytotoxic infusion of lung tumours.
3. Assessment of pulmonary atresia prior to surgery.

Technique

The bronchial arteries arise from the antero-lateral aspect of the proximal descending aorta. Variations are common but usually there are at least two arteries and in 20% of patients the left artery supplies a major branch to the spinal cord. For this reason the dose of contrast should be kept as small as possible and only non-ionic contrast (Iopamiro 300) should be used.

Catheter

A preshaped braided polyethylene 5.7F catheter is used. The tip configuration depends on the anatomy but a 'Cobra No. 2' or a 'Hilal Spinal' curve are usually satisfactory.

Technical problems

Unless they are large the bronchial arteries are not easily seen after aortic injections. A systemic catheter search is more rewarding. A subtraction of the left bronchial arteriogram should be viewed before embolization to exclude supply of the spinal cord.

Normally the injection of contrast will cause a cough reflex but most patients can overcome it and keep still.

Complications

Paraplegia may follow excessive contrast or emboli injected into the spinal artery.

Selective angiography of the subclavian artery branches

Indications

1. Selective angiography of the thyrocervical trunk and the internal mammary are necessary in parathyroid localization.
2. The costocervical trunk supplies branches to the spinal cord and should be avoided unless spinal angiography is required.
3. Selective injections of the other branches are sometimes indicated for the workup or embolization of vascular tumours, and in cases of severe chest wall trauma prior to embolization to control haemorrhage.

Catheter

A 5F polyethylene catheter is used as the arteries are small and wedging of larger catheters may occur. A short simple curve is made to suit the anatomy using boiling water to soften the catheter. If mini coils are to be used the polyethylene tubing should be 5.0 'M' not the usual 5.0 'B' (Cook Inc.) as the coils will jam in the thicker walled 'B' tubing.

Technical problems

A non-ionic contrast (Iopamiro) is used to reduce pain and in case of spinal cord supply. As the costocervical trunk and vertebral artery arise postero-superiorly from the subclavian artery they are usually the arteries entered most easily from below. The thyrocervical trunk and internal mammary arteries on the other hand arise antero-superiorly and often as a common trunk.

Complications

A subtracted angiogram should be performed prior to embolization of these arteries to ensure they do not contribute to the spinal or vertebral circulation.

Vena cavography

Inferior vena cava

Indications

1. Suspected thrombus in the IVC.

2. Assessment of renal tumours.
3. Budd–Chiari syndrome.

Patient preparation

As for aortography.

Technique

   1. Approach. Seldinger technique in common femoral vein on either side. The tip of the catheter is positioned at the conjunction of the common iliac veins.
   2. Catheter. A 6.5F polyethylene catheter 55 cm in length with 5 side holes near the tip.
   3. Wire guide. Teflon coated 'J-tip' with 1.5 mm curve radius 0.89 mm diameter.
   4. Site of injection. At the common iliac vein conjunction.
   5. Contrast. Iopamiro 370: 50–60 ml injected at 25–30 ml/s.
   6. Exposure sequence

[TIME (seconds)]
0 1 2 3 4 5 6 7 8 9 10 11 12 13 14 15 16 17 18 19
[INJECTOR]
★★★★
[EXPOSURE]
★★★★★ ★ ★
(3/s)

If the IVC is occluded a second slower injection may be required.

Equipment

Rapid film changer and automatic rate-controlled injector.

Technical problems

This examination is usually trouble free. A test injection should be made to exclude a large loose thrombus and to ensure that the catheter tip is not wedged in a lumbar vein. If the renal veins are not demonstrated a second injection with the patient performing a Valsalva manouvre may do so. Selective injections are required for opacification of the intro-renal veins. In Budd–Chiari syndrome caudate lobe hypertrophy will cause compression of the IVC but a catheter can usually be passed easily to the right atrium.

Complications

A loose thrombus may be dislodged by the catheter and a lumbar vein may be ruptured by a wedged injection. Both should be avoidable.

Superior vena cavography

Indications

1. Superior vena cava obstruction.
2. Assessment of extravascular shunts to the right atrium.

Parent preparation

Nil.

Technique

1. Approach. This examination may be performed in conjunction with an upper limb venogram or as a separate procedure. A catheter or a large bore needle is placed in the antecubital vein of one or both arms. If a catheter is used it should be advanced to the subclavian vein or innominate vein as indicated clinically.

2. Catheter. A 19 gauge scalp vein needle set or a 5F polyethylene catheter 55 cm in length with 5 side holes near the tip.

3. Wire guide. 'J-tip' with 1.5 mm curve radius 0.89 mm diameter and 80 cm in length.

4. Site of injection. See above.

5. Contrast. Iopamiro 370. A volume of 30 ml injected at 15 ml/s in each arm simultaneously. This requires two operators or a 'Y' piece connector for the injector. It is important that the patient does not hold his breath during the injection as this may cause spurious obstruction.

6. Exposure sequence

[TIME (seconds)]
0 1 2 3 4 5 6 7 8 9 10 11 12 13 14 15 16 17 18 19
[INJECTOR]
★★★★★
[EXPOSURE]
　　★　　★　　★　　★　　★　　　★

This series is designed to include the filling of the right and left heart as in cases of superior vena cava obstruction there may be occlusion of, or embolism of the pulmonary arteries.

Equipment

A rapid film changer is ideal but a spot film changer and a quick X-ray technician is an alternative.

Technical problems

When only one side is injected flow artefacts from the uninjected side may be confusing. Generally a bilateral injection is trouble-free.

Complications

Rare. See above.

Peripheral venography

Lower limb

Indications

1. Suspected venous thrombus.
2. Preoperatively for varicose veins.
3. Investigation of lower limb oedema.

Patient preparation

None required.

Technique

   1. Approach. Contrast is injected into a vein on the dorsum of the foot usually through a 19 or 21 gauge scalp vein needle set while a tourniquet is applied tightly just above the ankle. A cut-down is hardly ever required. If varicose veins are being studied further tourniquets are applied just below the position of the perforating veins. If both legs are to be studied examine one leg at a time. Place a step under the other leg so that the patient is raised on fluoroscopic table into a semi-erect position of about 60° and laid flat with the leg raised for the films of the pelvic veins. After the injection and filming is completed the leg should be exercised to remove contrast medium from the veins of the calf and lessen the chance of contrast-induced phlebitis.
   2. Contrast. A very large volume (150 ml) of diluted Angiografin 60 (diluted 1:1 with normal saline) injected by hand with three 50 ml syringes.
   3. Exposure sequence. The filling of the leg veins is monitored fluoroscopically and spot films made as the contrast progresses up the limb. The leg can be rotated if necessary to avoid overlap of vessels.

Technical problems

The most common problem is filling of the superficial veins only. This can be minimized by a more erect position and tighter tourniquets. The erect method fills all the available veins and the chance of a normal vein not filling is much less. The optimum time for the exposure is determined fluoroscopically. If the patient is unable to stand, undiluted contrast should be used.

Complications

High concentrations of contrast may cause a chemical phlebitis and produce thrombosis where none existed before the procedure. This effect is less likely if diluted contrast or non-ionic contrast is used (Albrechtsson 1979, Laerum & Holm 1981). It is theoretically possible to dislodge loose thrombi during the procedure. We have not seen a clinically evident example of this complication. The most common complication is extravasation of contrast at the injection site. If this occurs the injection should be stopped immediately. A warm towel placed over the extravasation may ease the patient's discomfort. Excessive extravasation of concentrated contrast may cause skin loss if the circulation is otherwise impaired.

Upper limb

Indications

1. Suspected venous thrombosis of the upper limb.
2. Investigation of upper limb oedema.

Patient preparation

Nil.

Technique

1. Approach. A 19 or 21 gauge scalp vein needle is inserted into a distal vein and contrast injected slowly preferably under fluoroscopic control. The site of obstruction (usually the axillary or subclavian vein) is identified and the time of optimum contrast opacification noted.

2. Contrast. Iopamiro 370. A hand injection of 25 ml at about 5 ml/s is sufficient.

3. Exposure sequence. The films are centred over the previously determined site of obstruction. The patient should not suspend respiration.

[TIME (seconds)]
0 1 2 3 4 5 6 7 8 9 10 11 12 13 14 15 16 17 18 19
[INJECTOR]
. (Hand)
[EXPOSURE]
    (At 2 second intervals from the time determined above)

Equipment

Angiographic or fluoroscopic room with spot film changer.

Technical problems

If the patient holds his breath a spurious obstruction may be seen. The fluoroscopic demonstration of the SVC filling is valuable as this technique will not completely opacify the SVC. In very fat patients streaming of contrast or partial compression of the axillary vein will be seen when the arm is abducted. In these cases the arm should be adducted to 90° and the contrast injection repeated.

Complications

Rare. See 'Superior venacavography'.

Pulmonary angiography

Indications

1. Acute pulmonary emboli prior to surgery or streptokinase.
2. To confirm a diagnosis of pulmonary embolism.
3. Diagnosis of pulmonary arteriovenous malformation.
4. Contraindication.
5. Severe pulmonary hypertension (PA Pressure > 90 mm Hg).

Patient preparation

Premedication with Atropine 0.6 mg. If the patient has pulmonary hypertension a separate IV line for the administration of inotropic agents is wise. Standard ECG monitoring is essential.

   In most cases anticoagulation can be continued especially if a cutdown approach is used. A femoral approach is only contraindicated if the bleeding time is more than 15 minutes.

Technique

   1. Approach. Either from the brachial vein (percutaneously or by cutdown) or from the femoral vein. Radiologists usually prefer the femoral route. From the femoral route almost all catheters will select the left pulmonary artery. If proceeding from the femoral route it is prudent to inject contrast under fluoroscopy as soon as the IVC is entered to exclude a thrombus in the IVC.

   2. Catheter. For most cases a braided polyethylene pigtail catheter with a 60° curve about 3 cm proximal to the pigtail (Grollman; Cook Inc.) is

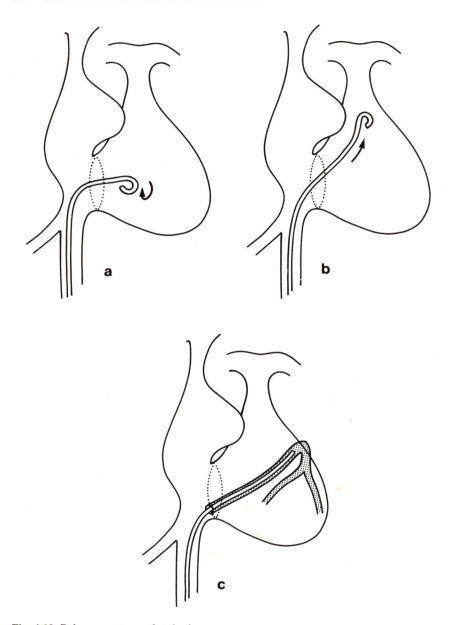

Fig. 4.12 *Pulmonary artery catheterization.*
(a) The catheter is inserted into the right ventricle. The pressure trace will indicate ventricular pressures. At a point close to the tricuspid valve the catheter is rotated so that the tip is directed upwards. (b) As the tip begins to point up the catheter is advanced gently towards the pulmonary valve. The catheter should cross the pulmonary valve easily and will usually enter the left pulmonary artery. (c) Incorrect placement of the catheter in the coronary sinus is detected by the low catheter position and the absence of a ventricular pressure trace.

adequate. This catheter is inserted with the Seldinger technique.

For more localized angiograms a closed end hole NIH catheter is used. This catheter also has a curved tip but the stiff end of the catheter is able to perforate the right ventricular outflow tract and should not be used by the inexperienced. The NIH catheter is introduced through a sheath.

Both catheters are introduced into the right ventricle and rotated to bring their tip upwards into the outflow tract of the right ventricle (see Fig. 4.12). The catheter is then advanced into the pulmonary artery. If resistance is felt or if a change in cardiac rhythm occurs the catheter should be withdrawn to the right atrium immediately.

3. Wire guide. A Teflon coated 'J-tip' with 1.5 mm curve radius 0.89 mm diameter is used for the initial catheterization. A deflecting tip wire guide may be necessary to turn the catheter from the left to the right pulmonary artery.

4. Site of injection. Contrast is injected into the main pulmonary artery on each side or more selectively as the circumstances dictate. If a massive pulmonary embolus has taken place a right ventricular injection may be all that is required.

5. Contrast. Iopamiro 370. Pulmonary artery injections make the patient cough particularly if large or if very selective. For the main pulmonary arteries 30–40 ml at 15–20 ml/s is required.

In cases of severe pulmonary hypertension a non-ionic contrast (Iopamiro) is indicated as they cause less elevation of the pulmonary artery pressure than ionic contrast.

6. Exposure sequence

[TIME (seconds)]
0 1 2 3 4 5 6 7 8 9 10 11 12 13 14 15 16 17 18 19
[INJECTOR]
****
EXPOSURE]
***** * *   *   *
(3/s)

Equipment

Catheter-tip pressure monitoring is essential and a pressure recorder is desirable. A rapid film changer and automatic rate-controlled injector are required.

Technical problems

A common problem is failure to enter the right ventricle particularly if the right atrium is dilated. Catheterization of the coronary sinus with the NIH catheter may cause an arrhythmia as indeed may catheterization of the right ventricle itself. If the pressure recorded is incompatible with the expected position of the catheter it should be withdrawn and the procedure tried again.

The NIH catheter may be curved in a hepatic vein and rotated as it is advanced into the right atrium. The pigtail catheter may be 'shaped' by bending the stiff end of the wire guide to the desired shape and inserting it stiff end first into the catheter. Under no circumstances should the stiff end of a wire guide protrude from the catheter.

The deflecting tip guide is used to turn the catheter from the left to the right main pulmonary artery. The catheter must be in the proximal portion of the main pulmonary artery before it is deflected. The catheter is then advanced off the wire guide.

Due to the proximal origin of the right upper lobe pulmonary artery, the catheter may recoil to the left if the catheter is positioned proximal to it. The right pulmonary artery injections should be made just distal to the upper lobe artery origin.

When small emboli are suspected many views and often selective magnified views may be necessary to exclude them. As the pulmonary pressure may rise significantly following contrast injections, the pressure should be monitored between injections.

If the patient coughs excessively the injected volume may be too high or the catheter may be partially wedged.

Complications

The major complication is perforation of the right ventricle with the catheter. If this is suspected do not perform a pericardiogram with contrast but aspirate the catheter as it is withdrawn to the right atrium. Monitor the pressure in the atrium and the systemic blood pressure in case pericardial tamponade develops. Pericardial aspiration may be necessary. In most cases, however, the pressure is low and the hole small so that the examination may proceed when the operator's tachycardia subsides.

Cor pulmonale may follow large injections of contrast in a patient with severe pulmonary hypertension. The patient may require removal of blood from the right heart while the left side should be stimulated with inotropes such as Isuprel in an infusion.

Contrast extravasation sometimes occurs after selective injections but is usually not serious and the contrast is rapidly absorbed unless a haematoma is produced. Sometimes a wedged injection is indicated to show the pulmonary veins in cases of anomalous venous return.

The occasional angiographer is advised to use digital subtraction angiography and atrial injections of Iopamiro 370 (40 ml at 15 ml/s).

PELVIC VENOGRAPHY

Indications

Diagnosis of pelvic vein thrombosis.

Patient preparation

Standard.

Technique

*1. **Approach.*** Both femoral veins are catheterized and using a 'loop catheter' technique the internal iliac veins are selectively catheterized.

*2. **Catheter.*** A 6.5F polyethylene catheter 65 cm in length with 5 side holes at the tip is used for each side. A braided catheter is usually not necessary and a 7–8 cm long curve may be placed in the catheter with boiling water. The catheters are joined with a 'Y' piece to the injector.

*3. **Wire guide.*** A teflon coated 'J-tip' with 1.5 mm curve radius 0.89 mm diameter and 145 cm in length for the insertion of both catheters.

*4. **Site of injection.*** The best position is usually just proximal to the confluence of the pelvic veins unless a more selective position is indicated on clinical grounds.

*5. **Contrast.*** Iopamiro 370. A volume of 50 ml is injected at 25 ml/s through the 'Y' piece to both catheters at once.

*6. **Exposure sequence***

[TIME (seconds)]
0 1 2 3 4 5 6 7 8 9 10 11 12 13 14 15 16 17 18 19
[INJECTOR]
★★★★★
[EXPOSURE]
★★★★★ ★ ★
(3/s)

Equipment

Rapid film changer and automatic rate-controlled injector.

Technical problems

Until the flow of blood can be reversed during life this examination will only demonstrate occlusion of the major veins. In most cases it is of limited clinical use. Often only the proximal portion of the major veins are opacified and the presence of pelvic vein thrombosis can neither be confirmed or denied.

Complications

It is possible to dislodge a loose thrombus with the catheter or the jet of contrast and to rupture the pelvic veins with injections of contrast through wedged catheters.

RENAL VENOGRAPHY

Indications

1. Demonstration of renal vein thrombosis.
2. Prolonged haematuria with a normal renal arteriogram.
3. The workup of renal tumours (occasionally).

Patient preparation

Standard.

Technique

1. Approach. Femoral vein using a 'loop catheter' technique as the catheter must be positioned to allow a high flow injection without recoil. Generally the loop will allow the catheter tip to be placed in the interlobular veins. In cases of nephrotic syndrome several selective injections may be required but the examination should start at the site of the renal biopsy if one has been performed.

2. Catheter. A 6.5F polyethylene non-braided catheter 65 cm in length with 5 side holes at the tip. A tight curve of 1–2 cm diameter is made 2–3 cm from the tip with boiling water for the right renal vein. The left renal vein often requires a wider curve of about 5 cm diameter in the same position. If the tip is too long or the curve too wide the catheterization may be difficult. When shaping catheters by hand it is easy to over-estimate the size of curve needed.

3. Wire guide. Teflon coated 'J-tip' with 1.5 mm curve radius 0.89 mm diameter and 145 cm in length. The wire guide is used to enter the IVC and if necessary the renal veins.

4. Site of injection. See 'Approach'.

5. Contrast. Iopamiro 370. A volume of 25 ml at 15 ml/s is injected.

6. Exposure sequence

[TIME (seconds)]
0 1 2 3 4 5 6 7 8 9 10 11 12 13 14 15 16 17 18 19
[INJECTOR]
∗∗∗∗
[EXPOSURE]
∗∗∗∗∗∗∗
(3/s)

Equipment

Rapid film changer and automatic rate-controlled injector.

Technical problems

Recoil of the right renal vein catheter may be impossible to prevent but positioning the catheter so that it is 'braced' against the opposite wall of the IVC may help. Sometimes the same shape will suit both renal veins. The 'right' shape described above is worth trying first for this reason.

A venous injection along is sufficient for workup of tumours and exclusion of major thrombi but if more detail of the small veins is required then the injection should be performed following renal artery injection of adrenaline. (This has been described in selective angiography.) The venous injection rate and volume is the same whether adrenaline is used or not. The venous injection should begin about 15–20 s after the adrenaline has been injected.

Complications

These are few. Extravasation of contrast is unusual and subclinical when it occurs. One serious problem is inadvertent catheterization of the left adrenal vein. A powerful injection in the adrenal vein may rupture it and cause necrosis of the gland.

A reasonable time should elapse between injections of adrenaline if it is being used.

RENAL VEIN SAMPLING

Samples of blood from the renal veins are required for renal vein renin estimations in the investigation of hypertension. The catheters are shaped as described for renal venography except that a single end hole catheter should be used.

As simultaneous samples are usually required both catheters are inserted in the same femoral vein but the second puncture is made either above or below the first. Take care not to puncture the first catheter with the needle for the second. Mark one of the catheters with an adhesive strip to avoid confusion as to which catheter is which and remove the sample syringes one at a time.

Generally venous angiograms and sampling may be performed on an outpatient basis provided the patient is not on anti-coagulants. After a period of about one hour of recumbency the patient is allowed to leave.

ADRENAL VENOGRAPHY AND VENOUS SAMPLING

Indications

This examination has been largely superseded by computed tomography but it is still used to localize the side of endocrine excretion particularly if the glands are hyperplastic.

Patient preparation

None required for the radiology but the endocrine service may require preparation to maximize the excretion of the hormone being sought.

Technique

1. Approach. Femoral vein puncture and selective catheterization of the adrenal veins bilaterally. The left drains into the left renal vein in most cases and is easy to catheterize especially with pre-shaped braided catheters. The right adrenal vein however is less constant and usually drains into the IVC directly at or above the level of the right renal vein. It is easy to confuse the small hepatic veins with the adrenal vein.

2. Catheter. Pre-shaped braided polyethylene 6.5F catheter 65 cm in length with a 'broad shepherds crook' curve at the tip. Alternatively a 'Cobra' shape or 'Sidewinder' shape may be used.

3. Wire guide. Teflon coated 'J-tip' with 1.5 mm curve radius 0.89 mm diameter 145 cm in length, and a Teflon coated straight 'long floppy' wire guide 0.89 mm diameter 145 cm in length for the selective catheterization.

4. Site of injection. Unless a venogram is indicated clinically only gentle hand injections are needed to confirm the catheter position. Wedged injections may rupture the adrenal vein.

5. Contrast. Angiografin 65. A total volume of 3–5 ml injected by hand.

6. Exposure sequence

[TIME (seconds)]
0 1 2 3 4 5 6 7 8 9 10 11 12 13 14 15 16 17 18 19
[INJECTOR]
HAND
[EXPOSURE]
***** * *
(3/s)

Technical problems

The major problem is inability to find the right adrenal vein. Rotating the patient to the right may profile the vein but IVC contrast injections are not helpful. When sampling the vein may collapse around the catheter if the catheter is forcibly aspirated. To avoid this cut a small 'v' in the end of the catheter or place a small side-hole very close to the catheter tip. The venous sampling should be performed slowly and gently as the venous outflow may be small.

Complications

The major complication is rupture of the adrenal vein and subsequent infarction of the adrenal gland.

SPLENO-PORTOGRAPHY

Indications

Diagnosis of portal hypertension.

This method has been used in the assessment of hepatic tumours but has been largely replaced by less invasive procedures.

In our institution this procedure has been replaced by selective high dose splenic arteriography and superior mesenteric arteriography. If portal venous pressures are required these are obtained indirectly from the hepatic venous pressure (see below).

Patient preparation

The patient should be fasted and the bowel cleared with aperients. A premedication is required. If there is evidence of severe liver dysfunction apiates should be avoided.

The bleeding and clotting times should be within normal range and a surgeon should be available for immediate laparotomy if required for haemorrhage.

Technique

1. Approach. The splenic position and size are determined with fluoroscopy or by skin markers and preliminary roentgenograms. Local anaesthetic injected into the skin and subcutaneous tissues is sufficient. In children a general anaesthetic is necessary.

With the patient supine a needle catheter combination is inserted to the expected region of the bilum of the spleen as determined above. The needle should be inclined slightly anteriorly to avoid the colon and pleural space. The needle catheter combination should enter the spleen at its closest point to the abdominal wall. Respiration should be as shallow as possible during the insertion.

When the needle is inserted to the desired position, the needle is withdrawn, leaving the catheter in position for injection of contrast. A free flow of blood indicates a correct position. At this time the splenic pulp pressure may be measured either by a vertical column of saline or strain-gauge manometry.

2. Catheter. A 19 gauge needle-cannula with Teflon sleeve catheter. These are listed by most manufacturers as splenoportogram needle-catheter sets.

3. Contrast. Iopamiro 370 is used for test injections under fluoroscopy before the patient is moved to a rapid film changer for the series. A volume of 50 ml injected at 8–10 ml/s is used for the examination. After the injection the catheter is removed. The patient should be kept under observation for 24–48 hours as late rupture of the spleen has been reported especially after subcapsular injections of contrast.

4. Exposure sequence. As usually only one injection is made the film programme should allow for all possibilities. This is not the time to economize on film.

[TIME (seconds)]
0 1 2 3 4 5 6 7 8 9 10 11 12 13 14 15 16 17 18 19
[INJECTOR]
****
[EXPOSURE]
* * * * * *   *   *   *   *   *   *   *

Equipment

Television fluoroscopy, a rapid film changer and automatic rate-controlled injector are required.

Technical problems

As the contrast is heavier than blood the posterior veins are opacified in preference to the anterior veins. This is most marked in the liver but it is not usually a diagnostic problem. In fact, it helps to localize the anatomic position of the veins.

If the test injection shows an unsatisfactory position the catheter should be repositioned. It is hazardous to insert the needle into the catheter while 'in situ' as the catheter may be transected by the needle tip.

If a satisfactory position has not been achieved after three or four punctures the examination should be postponed or an arterial indirect method used.

Occasionally the splenic blood may be diverted to a collateral circulation in the presence of a patent portal vein. In such cases the superior mesenteric vein should be studied either directly at surgery or indirectly by arteriography.

Complications

The most common complication is intro-abdominal haemorrhage which has in isolated instances caused death. Generally, haemorrhage producing clinical signs are rare.

Patients with aneurysms of the splenic artery near the splenic hilum are at increased risk of haemorrhage. As patients with portal hypertension and cirrhosis have an increased risk of splenic artery aneurysms arteriography has been suggested prior to spleno-portography.

Subcapsular or extrasplenic injections of contrast will cause pain of a severity and duration depending on the volume injected. Such pain may last for 6 to 8 hours.

Small intrasplenic aneurysms have been reported as a sequel to spleno-portography but they have been asymptomatic (Boijsen & Efsing 1967).

PARATHYROID VENOGRAPHY AND SAMPLING

Indications

Localization of parathyroid adenomata or hyperplasia.

The diagnosis of hyperparathyroidism is biochemical and venous sampling is usually only required after an initial operative removal of parathyroid glands has proved unsuccessful.

Patient preparation

A premedication containing opiates and diazepam is required as the examination is long and the X-ray table is uncomfortable. The patient will usually be aware of the catheters and wire guide manipulations in the neck veins.

In some cases where surgery has been performed more than once or in radical fashion the venous anatomy may be so disturbed that selective thyroid and internal mammary arteriography should be performed first to outline any anomalous veins (Doppman 1976).

Technique

1. Approach. Via the common femoral vein. Sampling the major veins is not sufficient as the right inferior thyroid vein may drain to the left innominate vein and mediastinal adenomata may drain to cervical veins and vice versa.

A forceful retrograde venous injection of contrast is made at the beginning of the procedure to provide a 'road map' to aid the examination and on which the site of each sample is recorded (see Fig. 4.13).

2. Catheter. A coaxial system is recommended as the normal anatomy is often disrupted by previous surgery. A 9F guide catheter 80 cm in length and an inner catheter of 5F polyethylene 100 cm in length is used with a torque control wire guide (Cook Inc.). In complicated cases a variety of shapes tailored to the veins at the time may be required. Alternatively more standard catheters may be used.

3. Wire guide. Teflon coated 'J-tip' with 1.5 mm curve radius 0.89 mm diameter 145 cm in length, and a Teflon coated straight 'long floppy' wire

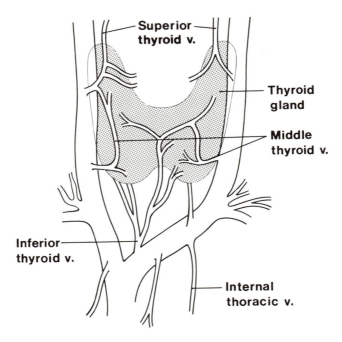

Fig. 4.13 *Schematic diagram of the thyroid veins.*
This or a similar diagram should be used to indicate the position of samples obtained during venous sampling for parathyroid tumours.

guide 0.89 mm diameter 145 cm in length for the selective catheterization. Deflecting tip wires and torque wires may also be required in difficult cases.

A fine gauge wire guide (0.45 mm diameter) is used with a Tuohy–Borst adapter to prevent the catheter tip obstructing on the vein wall when a sample is obtained.

4. Site of injection. The best single vein to make the injection of contrast in is the inferior thyroid vein especially if they form a single trunk. The middle thyroid veins are usually ligated at the first operation. The anterior jugular veins hardly ever drain parathyroid adenomata and should be avoided. More than one vein may need to be injected with contrast.

Samples should be obtained from both inferior thyroid veins as they are the normal drainage route for both the inferior and superior parathyroid glands. The middle thyroid, superior thyroid, vertebral, thymic and internal mammary veins on each side should be sampled if possible. At surgery many of these veins are ligated. The superior thyroid vein may drain into the facial vein. Samples from midline veins are not helpful in localizing adenomata. Samples from the innominate and internal jugular veins are included but are not often helpful in lateralization.

5. Contrast. Iopamiro 300. The volume and rate depend on the site of the injection and can be gauged from test injections. Hand injections are used for filming.

6. Exposure sequence. Usually a 100 mm camera is used at 2 exposures/s for 2–3 s.

Equipment

1. Television fluoroscopy.
2. Rapid film changer (100 mm camera is convenient).
3. Ice bucket for the blood samples.

Technical problems

Disturbed normal venous anatomy is the most common problem. Arterial studies may be necessary a few days before the venous sampling. When the catheter is in a small vein a forceful aspiration will cause the catheter to become impinged on the vein wall. A film run should accompany each sample to identify the sample position accurately. A very large dose of contrast may be used which may limit the length of the procedure. A urinary catheter may be required for the patient.

Complications

Rupture of veins or extravasation of contrast may occur but generally the examination is without incident.

TRANSHEPATIC VENOGRAPHY

Indications

1. Embolization of bleeding varices. (See Embolization, p. 135).
2. Venous sampling of the portal vein and its tributaries especially the pancreatic veins in endocrine tumour investigations.

Patient preparation

Standard premedication. The patient should be fasted and if the examination is elective or for sampling the bleeding and clotting times should be known.

Technique

1. Approach. The entry point is the right mid-axillary line just below the right costo-phrenic angle as determined fluoroscopically. Local anaesthetic is infiltrated into the skin subcutaneous tissues and down to the liver capsule. The needle is inserted towards a point about one vertebral body anterior to and to the right of the intervertebral space between the eleventh and twelfth thoracic vertebrae (see Fig. 4.14).

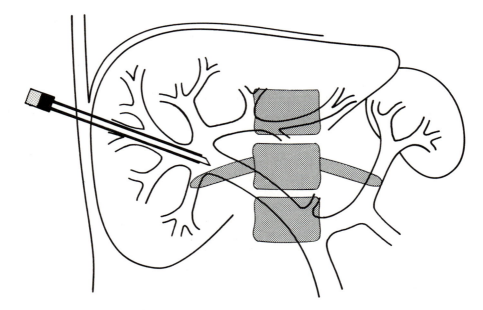

PANEL 1

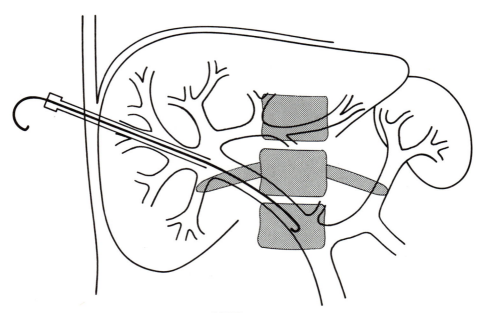

PANEL 2

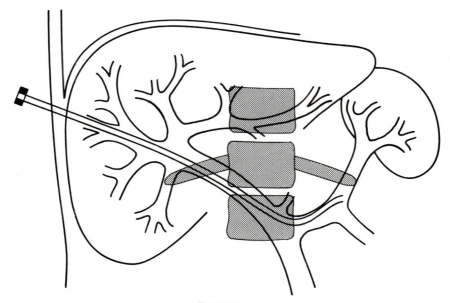

PANEL 3

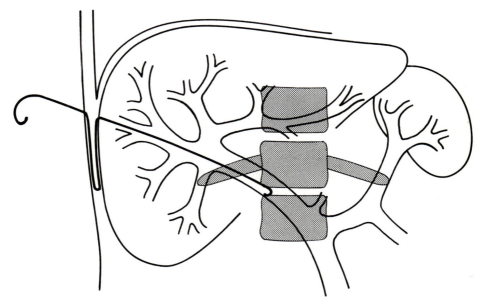

PANEL 4

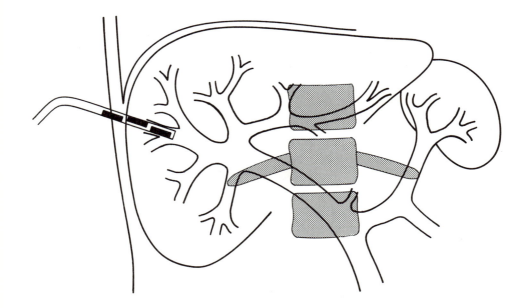

PANEL 5

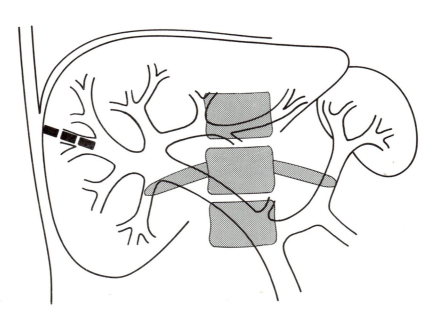

PANEL 6

2. Catheter. A 19 gauge needle 27 cm in length with a 5F polyethylene sheath is used for the puncture. The puncture is made with the patient in suspended quiet respiration. The needle is withdrawn and the catheter aspirated. When blood is aspirated contrast is injected to confirm the catheter is in a portal vein. A wire guide is inserted into the portal vein.

The 5F catheter may be exchanged over a wire guide with or without a vascular sheath for pre-shaped braided polyethylene catheters for more selective injections or embolization.

3. Wire guide. A Teflon-coated 'J-tip' with 1.5 mm curve radius 0.89 mm diameter and 145 cm in length is used to lead the polyethylene catheter into the main portal vein.

4. Site of injection. For most cases the injection should be made in the splenic vein close to the hilum of the spleen. Injections in the superior mesenteric vein or gastro-duodenal veins may be required prior to venous sampling. Bleeding varices should be injected with contrast before and after embolization.

Sampling requires a 'road map' and often considerable selective catheter work.

At the end of the procedure it is very important to embolize the tract from the liver capsule to the portal vein. This is accomplished with gelfoam 'torpedoes' (see Embolization below, p. 135) with a mini coil.

5. Contrast. Urografin 76. For the main veins 40 ml at 8–10 ml/s is sufficient. A slower rate should be used for selective injections of varices. Any gastric balloons for control of bleeding should be deflated before injection to allow the varices to fill with contrast.

6. Exposure sequence

[TIME (seconds)]
0 1 2 3 4 5 6 7 8 9 10 11 12 13 14 15 16 17 18 19
[INJECTOR]
****
[EXPOSURE]
 ★ ★ ★ ★★   ★   ★   ★   ★

Fig. 4.14 *Technique of transhepatic venography.*
Panel 1. A 19 gauge needle with plastic sheath is inserted into a large branch of the portal vein from the right side. *Panel 2.* After removal of the needle, a wire guide is inserted through the sheath and well down the portal vein. *Panel 3.* The sheath is exchanged for a catheter over the wire guide and advanced to the splenic vein. *Panel 4.* Avoid looping the wire guide between the skin and the liver capsule. Loops are produced by deep patient breathing or hard liver substance. A dilator may be required to straighten the wire.
Panel 5. The catheter track must be blocked with Gelfoam at the end of the procedure. Withdraw the catheter until it is almost out of the portal vein branch and then load several Gelfoam plugs into the catheter. *Panel 6.* Using a tuberculin syringe gently eject the plugs as the catheter is withdrawn. If they are soaked in contrast they will be visible for some minutes afterwards.

Equipment

1. Television fluoroscopy.
2. Rapid film changer.
3. Automatic rate-controlled injector.

Technical problems

If the portal vein is not cannulated the needle should be replaced inside the catheter without removing the catheter from the liver. Rotating the needle and re-inserting it under fluoroscopy will lower the likelihood of transecting the catheter. In most cases the portal vein can be entered within three passes of the needle. Sometimes the portal vein is not in the usual position and may be localized with ultrasound or arteriography.

If the liver is very cirrhotic or there is a large ascites the catheter will loop between the liver and the skin. The use of a stiffening cannual and a Teflon sheath will overcome this problem.

Complications

The major complication is bleeding from the puncture site in the liver. A small subcapsular haematoma is usual and blood may be found in the peritoneal space at surgery if performed soon after the transhepatic puncture.

The patient should be observed for 48 hours in case of significant blood loss. If the portal pressure is high and all the varices have been occluded completely there is a risk of portal vein thrombosis which is usually fatal. Such thrombosis is more likely if embolization has been repeated on several occasions.

Complications after sampling only are much less common.

LYMPHOGRAPHY AND LYMPH NODE BIOPSY

Indications

1. Demonstration of iliac and para-aortic lymphatics to stage cancer.
2. Investigation of lower limb oedema.
3. Investigation of filariasis, chylothorax and chyluria.
4. To check operative clearance of lymph nodes and to follow therapy by the means of follow-up films.
5. Lymphography is contraindicated in severe respiratory impairment or when there is skin sepsis.
6. Cervical and upper limb lymphography is of very limited application. These techniques are described elsewhere (Fuchs 1971).

Patient preparation

The examination is tedious and the patient should bring a book or other entertainment which will not cause his feet to move. The patient should be warned that the patent blue dye used in the examination will discolour his complexion for 12–24 hours and that his urine will be blue also. About 12 hours after the examination the contrast spills into the lungs and a slight fever or malaise is to be expected.

Technique

1. Approach. A patent blue dye is mixed with 1% local anaesthetic in equal parts and 1–2 ml of the mixture injected in the web-spaces between the first three toes of each foot. The feet are then exercised for a few minutes and the blue will outline the lymphatic channels on the dorsum of the foot. With full sterile precautions 1% local anaesthetic is injected intradermally and subcutaneously alongside a lymphatic on the mid-dorsum of one foot until a moderate lump is produced. An incision 1–2 cm long in the long axis of the foot is made directly over the lymphatic and extended to the subcutaneous tissues. The incision is quickly dissected with mosquito forceps and the lymphatic isolated with a short length of silk thread. If this is done quickly the lymphatic will be isolated before any bleeding obscures the wound. If the foot is massaged towards the wound the lymphatic should distend and the characteristic valves be identified.

The procedure is then repeated for the other foot.

2. Cannulation. Elevated by the silk thread, the lymphatic is gently stripped clean with a pair of fine tweezers. All fat must be removed from the lymphatic for about 2 cm. Rough treatment will rupture the lymphatic. A 25 or 30 gauge needle with tubing attached (Cook Inc.) is filled with saline and the tubing passed between two toes and secured with a gauze pad. A second silk thread is passed around the lymphatic and the first turn of a reef knot loosely made around the midportion of the lymphatic. The original silk thread is pulled tight in a cranial direction and fastened to the skin with adhesive tape.

The distal end of the lymphatic is retracted with straight tweezers and the needle bevel uppermost placed into the lymphatic as it leaves the tweezers. The needle is advanced and then, without releasing the tweezers, the second silk thread is gently tied around the needle close to the bevel. The lymphatic is released at each end and the adhesive tape used to secure the tubing close to the wound.

3. Injection. A test injection of saline is made and if there is no leakage, the first silk thread is also tied around the needle and lymphatic on the toe side of the bevel. This thread does not need to be very tight. Threaten the patient to keep still and warn him not to cross his legs as he relaxes.

Ultrafluid Lipiodol is the only oily contrast used but water soluble contrast such as Angiografin 65 may be used in cases of lymphoedema or when there is a possibility of direct venous injection.

A maximum of 10 ml of Ultrafluid Lipiodol is injected over 1.5–2 hours in each leg. The amount is reduced in small patients and in cases of respiratory disease.

A roentgenogram should be obtained of the pelvis and upper femora at 30 minutes after the injection starts to ensure there is no venous filling or abnormal lymphatico-venous communication. When the injection is completed the silk threads and needles are removed and if possible the lymphatic is preserved. Any oil should be washed from the wound and after an antibiotic spray the wound is sutured with an inverting mattress stitch.

4. Roentgenograms required. Exposures are made soon after the injection and about 24 hours later. Intravenous contrast may be given prior to the 24 hour-examination to determine the relationship of nodes to the renal tract. Antero-posterior and both oblique views of the abdomen, pelvis and upper femora, lateral views of the paraaortic nodes, an antero-posterior view of the thoracic spine, and an antero-posterior view of the lungs are required. Further localized or magnified views are obtained as indicated.

Equipment

Standard bucky radiographic table. Injector for lymphogram. The most satisfactory is simply a series of weights and a stand to hold them in position on the 10 ml syringes full of the contrast medium (Cook lymphographic injector).

Technical problems

In most cases lymphatics can be cannulated in 15–20 minutes but if they are small the procedure requires patience and a steady hand. If an assistant injects saline gently as the lymphatic is cannulated the lymphatic will distend and the insertion is easier. In the mid-dorsum of the foot there are several parallel lymphatics and if one is ruptured usually another can be found. Even if a second incision is required the foot does not look 'ring-barked' as it does with an extended transverse incision.

Small leaks of contrast may be ignored but large leaks require repositioning of the needle. The silk threads should be snug but able to be undone.

Complications

Allergic reactions to either oil or blue dye may occur but they are rare.

Wound infection or ascending lymphangitis may occur. Oily venous embolism occurs with all lymphography but if it occurs in large amounts it may cause pulmonary infarction and death.

Lymph node biopsy

This section refers to the percutaneous biopsy of lymph nodes using fluoroscopic guidance following lymphography (Gothlin & MacIntosh 1979).

Indications

1. Confirmation of equivocal metastatic disease on lymphography.
2. Staging of lymphomas and genitourinary cancer.
3. As an alternative to other more complicated types of biopsy for tissue typing of tumour, assessment of treatment or exclusion of lymphatic disease.

Patient preparation

Standard premedication.

Technique

1. Approach. The patient is biopsied in the supine position if possible with a vertically orientated needle.

The lymph nodes to be biopsied are localized fluoroscopically and after skin preparation, local anaesthetic is infiltrated into the skin, subcutaneous tissues and muscles. Avoid placing local anaesthetic near the lymph node as it distorts the cytology.

In very fat patients an 18 gauge needle 1.5 cm in length may be used to guide the finer aspiration needle through the skin. The aspiration is made with a 22 gauge Chiba needle 15 to 20 cm in length.

2. Biopsy. The 22 gauge needle is introduced under fluoroscopic control until the tip of the needle is directly over the suspect area of the lymph node. As the needle is advanced the lymph node will be displaced, distorted and finally with a slight loss of resistance, be punctured by the needle. This procedure is much easier with bi-plane fluoroscopy but rotating the patient or wobbling the needle from side to side will also confirm correct placement.

While suction is applied the needle is moved up and down slightly for 10–15 seconds. The suction is released and the needle withdrawn. Smears of the material are made immediately on glass slides for examination. The patient is kept in the room until the cytologist determines that lymphatic tissue is present. This takes about 10 minutes if the cytologist is present.

Equipment

Facilities for a rapid Papanicolaou stain, a microscope and cytologist in the X-ray room reduce the time for this procedure and repeat biopsies can be performed if necessary without delay. Biplane fluoroscopy is not essential but very useful.

Technical problems

The major problem is an unrepresentative sample. In practice the correlation between aspiration biopsy and histology of surgically removed nodes is high.

If the nodes lie close to the IVC blood may contaminate the sample. The aorta is less readily punctured inadvertently. If a nerve bundle is punctured the patient will complain of radiating severe pain. Biopsy in this situation has caused temporary difficulty in walking.

The only contraindication is a severe bleeding tendency.

Complications

The procedure is usually performed on an outpatient basis. There is a risk of seeding of tumour along the aspiration track with large bore needles but with 22 gauge or smaller needles there have been only two documented cases in over 6000 percutaneous biopsies (Ferrucci et al 1979, Sinner & Zajicek 1976).

Although the bowel is often perforated by the needle we have seen no sequelae related to this. The needle track is almost impossible to find at surgery. A small haematoma may occur in the abdominal wall but generally the procedure is well tolerated and similar in discomfort level to a venupuncture (Antonovic et al 1976).

DIGITAL SUBTRACTION ANGIOGRAPHY

Introduction

Digital subtraction angiography is the application of computer technology to a long standing practice of 'analogue subtraction' of pre- and post-contrast images to enhance contrast and remove unwanted information present on the pre- and post-contrast images.

The advantages of the 'digital subtraction' are faster diagnosis, less contrast medium is required (for arterial studies), less catheter skills are required, and less cost particularly in film costs and room usage. The procedure is safer for the patient and is an outpatient procedure in most cases.

The disadvantages are the large doses of contrast required (for intravenous studies), motion artefacts, and the overlap of vessels when intravenous injections of contrast are used.

It is very easy to use excessive numbers of exposures and the radiation dose received by the patient may be high.

Arterial studies

The dose of contrast may be reduced to 50% or less of that for standard examinations. The same volume should be used to avoid mixing artefacts.

In some cases full strength contrast may be required for test injections as the diluted contrast may not be dense enough for fluoroscopy.

The contrast should be diluted with water for injection but solutions hypontonic with respect to the blood should not be used.

The same film programs should be used as for standard studies. Often less selective injections are required and this together with the lower dose of contrast and shorter time for the examination increase patient safety.

Intravenous studies

Full strength contrast (Iopamiro 370) is injected rapidly into a central vein or the right atrium and a series of exposures made of the area to be examined at a time after the injection consistent with the distance from the heart and the speed of the circulation.

Peripheral injections produce a less cohesive bolus, the peak concentration of contrast is lower, and the diagnostic quality lower than with central injections.

We recommend a commercial set (DSAY RMH: Cook Inc.) which starts with a 21 gauge needle and results in a 5F polyethylene catheter 55 cm in length with 5 side holes at the tip being placed in the right atrium. Larger catheters may be used but we have not found them necessary and they cannot be used when the arm veins are poor.

Patients with poor arm veins have a femoral vein catheter inserted instead. This is also done as an outpatient using the 5F catheter as above.

Procedure

The area to be examined is positioned with fluoroscopy and the image smoothed by added filtration. We use magnetic rubber sign material of various shapes applied to the face of the collimator. These may be shaped with a pair of scissors and are inexpensive. Added filtration is required in thin body parts adjacent to thicker parts because of the limited dynamic range of the image camera.

Immobilization

Motion artefacts are caused by respiratory excursion, swallowing or conscious movements and sometimes by the sudden onset of the sensation of heat produced by the contrast causing motion of the head or limbs. An interpreter is required if there is a language incompatibility.

For carotid studies the head is strapped into a foam pad and the patient instructed carefully to hold their breath and not to swallow when the injection starts. They are also told what to expect from the contrast injection. The importance of immobility is explained to the patient. These steps are conveniently practised while the operator is inserting the catheter.

Abdominal studies require compression and paralysis of the bowel with either Buscopan or glucagon given just before the injection of contrast. Alternatively, a 'dual energy' hybrid subtraction method may be used if one has the necessary equipment.

Contrast injection

A volume of 30–40 ml of Iopamiro 370 is injected at 15–20 ml/s. The contrast reaches the arch of the aorta 3–4 s after the start of injection, the carotid bifurcation and renal arteries at 4–8 s after the start of the injection and the common femoral artery at 10–12 s after the start of the injection in normal individuals using a 5F right atrial catheter. There is no evidence that any one contrast is superior in achieving better contrast in digital subtraction angiography than any other but preference should be given to agents which cause the least patient intolerance and least effect on cardiovascular function. In our experience the incidence of reactions to contrast is extremely low and less than for urography. The reasons for this are not clear.

Exposures are made in three groups: the first group of 3 at 1/s, the second group at 2–3/s for 6–8 s and the last group of 4 at 1/s. The exposure sequence is terminated as soon as the contrast bolus has disappeared. The timing is arranged so that the bolus arrives as the rapid exposure sequence starts.

Complications

In 900 examinations we have had one serious complication. A patient with heart disease developed heart failure due to fluid overload and suffered a major myocardial infarction. Venous extravasation has occurred infrequently and has been clinically asymptomatic. Patients with angina may develop chest pain after the third or fourth injection. In such cases the examination is terminated or truncated.

Uncooperative patients or those with severe Parkinson's disease are not suitable for the intravenous method. If the cardiac output is poor the contrast will be poor and a diagnostic study may not be possible.

INTERVENTIONAL RADIOLOGY TECHNIQUES

Interventional radiology is an extension of the diagnostic techniques to the treatment of disease processes. They are surgical in effect but for the size of the incision required and the complications may be major. They should not be attempted by those without specialized training and they should not be performed in isolation as the complications may require urgent surgical or medical intervention.

Angioplasty

Indications

1. Any discrete stenosis or short occlusion in an accessible artery with good distal vessels.
2. Selected cases with a localised proximal stenosis but poor distal vessels when used for limb salvage or to aid healing of an ischaemic ulcer.
3. Angioplasty of the internal carotid artery carries an unacceptable risk of stroke.
4. Vascular surgical support should be available.

Technique

The patient is often placed on anti-platelet medication (Aspirin) prior to the procedure and in the case of coronary angioplasty a nitroglycerine infusion is performed during the dilation. Cardiac monitoring and pressure monitoring is used for coronary and renal angioplasty but not usually for femoral or iliac angioplasty.

If a sheath or coaxial guide catheter is used the stenos may be localized by contrast injections but if not the stenosis is marked with an artery clip on the drapes. Parallax error will occur if the image intensifier is moved.

A wire guide is passed under fluoroscopic control across the stenosis or occlusion and the angioplasty catheter positioned in the narrowed segment. Before the balloon is inflated the catheter should be aspirated or contrast injected to ensure that the tip is still in the lumen. This is very important if an occluded segment is to be dilated.

The balloon is inflated slowly with diluted contrast using a pressure gauge to its maximum diameter in one or in several inflations and an angiogram performed to assess the dilatation.

If there are several stenoses the most distal one is dilated first and the wire guide should be left across the stenoses during the angioplasty.

The angioplasty will produce a sensation of pressure during inflation of the balloon which usually indicates a satisfactory dilatation. Severe pain indicates a dilated dissection.

Anticoagulants are generally used (heparin 5000 IU) except for some femoral dilatations when the procedure will be very short.

1. Catheter. The diameter of the balloon should be commensurate with the size of the artery to be dilated. In general 2.5–3.0 mm diameter balloons are used for coronary arteries, 9–10 mm diameter balloons for iliac arteries and 5–6 mm diameter balloons are used for renal and femoral arteries.

The most convenient balloon lengths are 2–4 cm. The French size of the angioplasty catheter is determined by the size of the balloon.

The easiest catheters to use inflate and deflate quickly and have a low profile of the balloon on the shaft so that they are easy to pass across narrowed areas and will not cause leakage around the catheter at the puncture site. (Cook Dotter or Omega angioplasty.)

If the angioplasty is to be performed with access through a dacron graft a sheath is necessary to avoid damage to the balloon catheter.

2. Wire guide. Teflon coated 'J-tip' with 1.5 mm curve radius 0.89 mm diameter and 145 cm in length to enter the artery and a Teflon coated 'long (10 cm) floppy tip' 0.89 mm diameter and 145 cm in length to cross the stenosis. For occlusions a straight wire with a non-tapered mandrel or a stiffening cannula may be used. (GRM: Cook Inc.)

Technical problems

It may be difficult to localize short stenoses in the renal or iliac arteries as they change position with wire guides or the catheters in them. A long balloon will overcome this.

A distal renal artery stenosis may not provide room for the tip of the angioplasty catheter beyond the stenosis without wedging the catheter. These need careful dilatation and flushing of the catheter as soon as possible after the distal lesion has been dilated. For flushing the catheter may need to be withdrawn.

With popliteal arteries ensure that the catheter is not in a geniculate branch as dilatation of such a branch may occlude the popliteal artery just beyond the branch origin.

If the balloon will not deflate it may be punctured percutaneously but persistent aspiration with a large volume syringe usually prevails. Do not withdraw an inflated balloon from the artery.

Avoid angioplasty of acutely occluded segments unless any fresh thrombus has been cleared by thrombectomy or streptokinase.

Complications

Any complication of angiography may occur. A certain amount of embolization is common but usually this is not significant. The artery may occlude as a result of prolonged spasm or dissection. Long stenotic segments in narrow arteries are prone to early occlusion and are best avoided.

Haematomata are fairly common due to the anticoagulation and the large size of many of the catheters.

Rupture of the renal artery during angioplasty has been reported. Inflation of the balloon in the arterial stump should arrest the blood loss but acute surgery will be needed to save the kidney.

Immediate surgical backup is also required for coronary angioplasty.

Trans-catheter embolization

Indications

1. Control of haemorrhage.
2. Reduction of arterial supply pre-operatively.
3. Palliation of tumours.
4. Obliteration of arterio-venous fistulae.

Patient preparation

The embolization may produce severe pain in the target area and an opiate containing premedication is required. Informed consent is essential.

Antibiotic prophylaxis with Gentamicin and Amoxicillin is recommended to prevent infection of the infarcted tissue. Embolization of the spleen must be performed in small stages as total embolization is invariably associated with sepsis even with antiobiotics.

Material used

For short term occlusion: Gelfoam (Upjohn)
Permanent occlusion: Coils (Cook)
                              Ivalon particles (Unipoint)
Arterio-venous fistulae: De Brun Detachable Balloons (Ingenor)
                              Isobutyl Cyanacrylate (Ethnor)
Renal tumours, varices: Absolute alcohol

This is a short list. Materials from blood clot to aqueous Dionosil and most recently lasers have been used.

Technique

Gelfoam is used as shavings or chunks cut with a scalpel or scissors and injected in a slurry of saline or contrast. A small (2 ml) syringe should be used to avoid recoil of the catheter from excessive pressures. If the catheter becomes blocked and it is still in a safe position, clear it with a wire guide and a tuberculin syringe. Larger pieces if cut on a taper can be rolled tightly to form 'torpedoes' which expand on entering the artery. They are loaded one per syringe (2 ml) with the tip just protruding from the syringe. Start with small pieces and end with a big piece.

Coils are wire guide spirals with dacron threads at right angles to the spiral core. They come in three sizes and are loaded into the catheter from a metal sleeve with the stiff end of wire guide. The wire guide should be passed through the catheter first to ensure that the catheter will not become dislodged when the coil is delivered. Arteries may recannalize centrally if the coil lies in a position at right angles to the long axis of the artery and they are best avoided if repeated embolization is thought to be necessary.

Ivalon sponge particles are polyvinyl alcohol particles available in graded sizes. They are sterilized as needed by autoclave in a small dish containing a little water. The resulting slurry is diluted further and the particles loaded by aspiration into a 2 ml syringe. The particles settle from the suspension quickly and are agitated immediately before injection. Large quantities will clog the catheter. The particles are impregnated with barium and form an arterial cast.

Detachable balloons are flow guided and used mostly for carotico-cavernous fistulae. Their use is beyond the scope of this book.

Cyanoacrylate is not an approved substance for general use. It is usually opacified with tantalum powder and retarded with Pantopaque (Myodil). Cyanoacrylate is delivered via a coaxial catheter system flushed with dextrose to avoid premature polymerization. The delivery catheter is with-drawn at the end of injection to avoid being trapped in the polymer. An occluding balloon catheter may be used to control blood flow and over-penetration of the polymer.

Absolute alcohol is delivered with a flow-directed occlusion balloon cath-eter (Meditech Inc.) to control blood flow and prevent entry of the alcohol to the rest of the circulation. The injection of alcohol is initially very painful but it appears to cause less pain afterwards. A volume of 5–10 ml is infused while the balloon is inflated. After 1–2 minutes the balloon is slowly deflated and contrast injected to ensure the vessels are occluded.

Complications

Embolization of unwanted vessels is the major complication. This usually results from dislodgement of the catheter, or from washout of emboli from the target vessel. It is prudent to stop the embolization as soon as the flow effectively stops as the normal clotting processes will complete the occlu-sion.

Nerve injury will follow the use of liquids or very fine particles for embolisation. The sciatic nerve (pelvic embolization) and the facial nerve (external carotid embolization) are the most common nerves injured in this way.

Vaso-constrictor infusions

Indications

1. Control of bleeding when embolization is contraindicated.
2. Enhancement of tumour circulation.

Technique

Enhancement of tumour circulation with adrenaline is described in the section on renal arteriography (p. 90) and coeliac arteriography (p. 93).

Variceal bleeding may be effectively controlled by intravenous as arterial infusions.

For control of bleeding vasopressin is infused through a selectively placed catheter after an arteriogram has demonstrated the site of bleeding.

1. Titration. A dose of 0.05 to 0.1 units/minute is infused for 15 minutes and the arteriogram is gently repeated with a slower rate of injection to document control of bleeding. If bleeding is not controlled the catheter should be positioned closer to the bleeding site or the dose increased. After a further 20 minutes the arteriogram is repeated.

2. Infusion. The infusion is continued at the control rate for 24 hours and at half the control rate for a further 24 hours. If the dose was very low (<0.05 units/minute) the catheter can be removed, but if control was difficult the catheter should be left in situ and saline infused for a further 24 hours in case of recurrence of bleeding.

If bleeding occurs the catheter position should be checked before the infusion rate is increased.

3. Mixtures and equipment. If the saline infusion rate is 50 ml/hour, and the vasopressin dose 0.05 units/minute, then a 500 ml bottle of saline requires 30 units for the correct mixture. A dose over 1.0 units/minute, will produce systemic effects of pallor, sweating, and sometimes angina pectoris.

Our infusion patients are cared for in the intensive care unit while vasopressin is running. During the infusion the patient's serum electrolytes and fluid balance should be monitored and if it is available they should be on cardiovascular monitoring. A confusional state may indicate hyponatraemia and/or cerebral oedema.

Technical problems

For the easiest control of the infusion rate a drip fed syringe actuated delivery system with a 10–12-hour 'range' is desirable. A suitable type is illustrated (see Fig. 4.15). The flow rate should be high enough to keep the catheter patent. For a 6.5F catheter this requires about 50 ml/hour.

The catheter should be sutured to the skin in a loop so that if the ignorant bystander should pull on the catheter it will not be dislodged. Inspection of the puncture site should only be performed when the radiologist is present.

When the catheter is removed it will be coated in fibrin and blood clot which may be stripped off as the catheter is withdrawn. Pressure should not be applied to the artery until the catheter is out and the catheter should be aspirated by an assistant during removal.

Complications

Complications are dose-related and if major complications arise the infusion should be discontinued. Major complications include cerebral oedema,

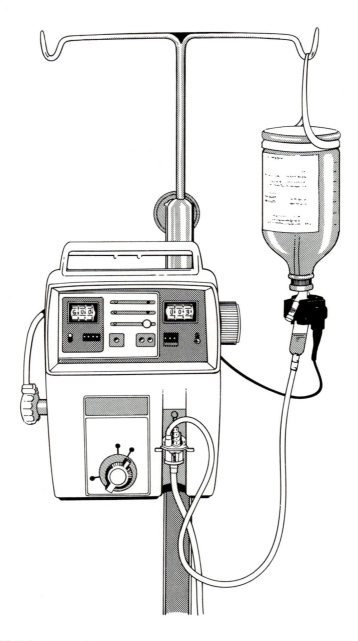

Fig. 4.15 *Infusion pump for arterial infusions.*
This unit uses a small pumping chamber and delivers a pulsed flow at rates up to 15 ml/minute. It has built-in alarms for injection of air, and blockage of the flow. The unit keeps a record of the volume delivered and has a volume limit which can be set up to 1 l.

myocardial infarction, and infarction of the bowel. Minor complications include hyponatraemia, cardiac arrhythmias, oliguria and peripheral acrocyanosis.

Cytotoxic infusion

Indications

Cytotoxic drug infusion offers the promise of better palliation of cancer with reduced side effects because the drug is delivered at the site of the tumour. In fact, there is no evidence from controlled trials to support this promise and the technique is only practised in certain centres.

Technique

A catheter is placed usually from the axilla to allow the patient mobility during the term of the infusion. An infusion pump similar to that described above for vasopressin is generally used but for very long-term infusions portable or implantable pumps have been devised.

If the target organ is supplied by several arteries the blood supply may be altered by embolization to provide only one artery of supply. This is most commonly performed in infusion of liver tumours.

At the end of the infusion if it has not already occluded the artery may be embolized.

Technical problems

If the catheter becomes dislodged the drug may cause untoward side effects. The tumour effect is not altered much as the drug is always present systemically no matter where it is delivered. A hepatic infusion which becomes dislodged and infuses the stomach instead will cause nausea and pain each time the infusion is started. The best way to assess the area infused is to inject an isotope at the perfusion rate and image the patient.

There is a direct relationship between the length of perfusion and the catheter related complications. The catheter is anchored as for vasopressin infusions. If the catheter needs to be changed an exchange guide is used and the catheter thoroughly soaked in alcoholic chlorhexidine but the skin cannot be sterilized to a bacteriologist's satisfaction.

Complications

Fracture of the catheter and leakage around the puncture site are common and false aneurysm formation or loss of the radial pulse have been recorded (Clouse et al 1977).

These have complications which have not provided sufficient contraindications to the use of the brachial route and compared to the alternative femoral or direct surgical routes the complications are reasonable. A large number of catheters occlude with thrombus and many infused arteries thrombose also.

The complications listed above for axillary punctures also apply.

Removal of clotted catheter

Introduction

If a catheter becomes occluded with thrombus and the examination is finished then no problem exists.

If blood cannot be aspirated through the catheter then there are several possibilities. Check the position of the catheter to ensure it is not wedged or pointing at the arterial wall and withdraw it aspirating as you do so. Check the length of the catheter to ensure that it has not kinked or twisted (usually in the iliac artery) during a difficult examination. If this is the problem insert a wire guide and unwind the catheter under fluoroscopy taking care not to tighten any knot.

Knots are best avoided as they are impossible to untie if they have been drawn tight. In this situation pull the knot to the femoral puncture site and call your vascular surgeon. If he is unavailable most tightly knotted catheters may be wrenched out of the puncture site but at the risk of severe damage to the artery and false aneurysm.

Catheters occluded with fresh clot will usually clear with strong aspiration. Never be tempted to pass a wire guide or flush the clot out as it may be quite large.

Preferred method

Withdraw the catheter below the renal arteries and with a scalpel cut a side hole in the catheter about 10 cm from the skin entry. Take care that the hole does not weaken the catheter unduly. If blood pours out a wire guide can be inserted safely and the clotted catheter changed over the wire guide.

If no blood pours out, the tip of the catheter is clotted. Insert a 3 mm 'J-tip' wire guide stiff end first into the side hole in the direction of the tap end of the catheter until the soft tip of the wire guide is flush with the catheter. Check that the wire guide will advance out the side hole and if so, insert the catheter with the wire guide flush into the artery until the side hole is 10 cm up the artery.

The wire guide is then advanced out the side hole for 30–40 cm and the catheter withdrawn from the artery leaving the wire guide in the artery. A new catheter is replaced over the wire guide.

Alternative method

The clotted catheter is cut across 20 cm from the skin and a close fitting sheath passed over the catheter into the artery. The catheter is then replaced via the sheath. This method sounds easy but in practice the sheath usually buckles and insertion is often difficult or impossible.

Removal of catheter and wire guide fragments from the circulation

For the capture and removal of catheter and wire guide debris either a multiwired Dormier basket or a wire snare is used. A simple method is a combination of a 6.5F braided polyethylene catheter with a 'Cobra No. 2' curve to give directional control and an exchange wire guide 260 cm long and 0.46 mm diameter (0.018 in) to form the snare. The mid-point of the wire guide is crimped in a pair of artery forceps and the wire guide inserted through the catheter. As it emerges the crimped end causes the two halves of the wire guide to part and form a loop which is tightened by pulling on the two ends of the wire guide. Holding one end fixed and retracting the other causes the loop to deviate to the retracted side.

The loose fragment is manipulated into the loop and when tightly caught withdrawn to the puncture site. The site of puncture depends on the site of the embolus. In our experience most emboli are non-opaque central venous catheters which are lodged in the heart or pulmonary arteries. Often the fragments are caught on a trabeculum and may be difficult to catch in the snare. Many are pushed further downstream during the retrieval.

Intentional abuse of a wire guide for this method is not condoned by the manufacturer.

REFERENCES

Adams D F, Fraser D B, Abrams H L 1973 The complications of coronary arteriography. Circulation 48: 609–618

Albrechtsson U 1979 Side effects at phlebgraphy with ionised and non-ionised contrast medium. Diagnostic Imaging 48: 236–240

Ansari Z, Baldwin D S 1976 Acute renal failure due to radio contrast agents. Nephron 17: 28–40

Antonovic R, Rosch J, Dotter C T 1976 Complications of percutaneous transaxillary catheterization for arteriography and selective chemotherapy. Radiology 126: 386–393

Boijsen E, Efsing H O 1967 Intrasplenic arterial aneurysms following splenoportal phlebography. Acta Radiologica (Diagnostica) 6: 487–496

Brash R C 1980 Allergic reactions to radiographic contrast media: accumulated evidence. American Journal of Roentgenology 134: 797–801

Clouse M E, Ahmed R, Ryan R B, Oberfield R R, McCaffrey J A 1977 Complications of long term transbrachial hepatic arterial infusion therapy. American Journal of Roentgenology 129: 799–803

Doppman J L 1976 Parathyroid localization: arteriography and venous sampling. Radiologic Clinics of North America 2: 163–188

Ferrucci J T, Wittenburg J, Margolies N M 1979 Malignant seeding of the tract after thin-needle aspiration biopsy. Radiology 130: 345–346

Fischer H W, Thomson K R 1978 Contrast media in coronary arteriography: a review. Investigative Radiology 13: 450–459

Fuchs W A 1971 Technique and complications of lymphangiography. In: Abrams H L (ed.) Angiography. 2nd edn. Little, Brown, Boston. pp 1325–1335

Gothlin J H, MacIntosh P K 1979 Interventional radiology in the assessment of the retroperitoneal lymph nodes. Radiologic Clinics of North America 17: 461–473

Greitz T, Lindgren E 1971 Cerebral angiography; techniques and hazards. In: Abrams H L (ed.) Angiography. 2nd edn. Little, Brown, Boston. pp 155–168

Hessel S J, Sequira J C 1981 Femoral artery catheterization and vessel tortuosity. Cardiovascular and Interventional Radiology 4: 80–82

Johnsrube I S, Jackson D C 1979 A practical approach to angiography. Little, Brown, Boston.

Judkins M P 1967 Selective coronary arteriography–1: a percutaneous transfemoral technic. Radiology 89: 815–824

Kallenhauge H E, Praestholm J 1982 Iopamidol, a new non-ionic contrast medium in peripheral angiography. Cardiovascular and Interventional Radiology 5: 325–328

Laerum F, Holm H A 1981 Postphlebographic thrombosis: a double-blind study with methylglucamine metrizoate and metrizamide. Radiology 140: 651–654

Lalli A F 1980 Contrast media reactions: data analysis and hypothesis. Radiology: 137–869

Michels N A 1955 Blood supply and anatomy of the upper abdominal organs. Lippincott, Philadelphia. pp 152–154, 256–259, 374–375

Older R A, Korobkin M, Cleeve D M, Schaaf R, Thompson P 1980 Contrast induced renal failure: persistent nephrogram as a clue to early detection. American Journal of Roentgenology 134: 339–342

Sage M R, Drayer B P, Dubois P J 1981 Increased permeability of the blood–brain barrier after Renografin-76. American Journal of Neuroradiology 2: 272–274

Shehadi W H, Toniolo G 1980 Adverse reactions to contrast media (A report from the Committee on Safety of Contrast Media of the International Society of Radiology). Radiology 137: 299–302

Sigstedt B, Lunderquist A 1978 Complications of angiographic examinations. American Journal of Roentgenology 130: 455–460

Sinner W N, Zajicek J 1976 Implantation metastasis after percutaneous transthoracic needle aspiration biopsy. Acta Radiologica (Diagnostica) 17: 473–480

Spigos D G, Akkinei S, Tan W, Espinoza D A, Flanigan D P, Winnie A 1980 Epidural anaesthesia: effective analgesia in aorto-ilio-femoral arteriography. American Journal of Roentgenology 134: 335–337

Tress B M, Field P 1981 'A hair's breadth away'. Australasian Radiology 25 (1): 13–15

Thomson K R, Schering A G 1987 Iopamiro in reactors. Australasian Iopamidol Trials

Yocum M W, Heller A M, Abels R I 1978 Efficacy of intravenous pre-testing and antihestamine prophylaxis in radio-contrast media-sensitive patients. Journal of Allergy and Clinical Immunology 62: 309–313

5

Cerebral angiography

INTRODUCTION

With the development of alternative imaging techniques, such as computed tomography (CT) and magnetic resonance imaging (MRI), the originally broad applications of cerebral angiography have become much more narrow and defined. The principal indications for cerebral angiography are:
1. Transient ischaemic attacks, including vertebrobasilar insufficiency (VBI).
2. Determination of aetiology of subarachnoid haemorrhage.
3. Pre-operative 'road map' prior to tumour surgery.
4. Suspected cerebral arteritis.
5. Establishment of route for embolization of fistulae, vascular malformations and tumours.
6. Diagnosis of traumatic and spontaneous dissection of major cerebral blood vessels.

METHODS

The standard cerebral studies are common carotid and vertebral selective angiograms and non-selective arch aortography. All are usually performed with catheters via one or other common femoral artery. Only extremely rarely, such as in the absence of femoral pulses, must direct carotid or vertebral punctures be attempted. With the advent of the less invasive technique of intravenous digital subtraction angiography (IV DSA) transaxillary or transbrachial approaches for vertebral angiography are virtually procedures of last resort. The external carotid artery and each of its branches may be selectively catheterized via the transfemoral approach.

MATERIALS

Catheters

A large number of catheter materials, shapes and sizes have been described. Virtually all cerebral vessels may be safely negotiated by one or other of the following four catheter types:

143

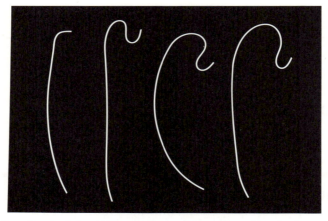

Fig. 5.1 5 French polyethylene 140 cm catheters. From left to right the shapes are designed for patients up to 20 years old, 20–40, 40–60 and greater than 60 years old, respectively.

1. 5 French polyethylene (PE) 140 cm. This relatively atraumatic, slightly tapered catheter is the basic catheter for most standard studies, as well as the ideal catheter for superselective external carotid artery branch arteriography (Fig. 5.1). It can be purchased preshaped, or may be shaped prior to use over a steam jet, or in boiling water.
2. 5 French PE, 'Mani' catheter (Mani 1970). Its preshaped acute curve is particularly suitable for the acutely angled takeoff of left common

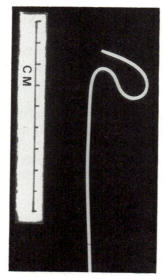

Fig. 5.2 5 French polyethylene 'Mani' catheter.

carotid artery from aortic arch in middle-aged, elderly and hypertensive patients, but it is less suitable for use in young patients (Fig. 5.2).

3. Simmons 'Sidewinder' catheter (USCI), (Simmons et al 1973). The 7 French diameter of most of the length of this catheter allows excellent torque control from manipulation at the groin, while abrupt tapering of its terminal 8 cm to 5 French allows it to be manipulated in the proximal common carotid artery without a guidewire (Fig. 5.3). It is particularly suitable for the elongated aortic arches of atheromatous patients.

4. Berenstein 'Hockey Stick' catheter (USCI). As with the Simmons catheter, only the terminal 10 cm is tapered to 5 French, allowing excellent, relatively safe manipulation of the catheter within the cerebral vessels of adolescents and adults of all ages (Fig. 5.4). It may even be used for superselective studies of external carotid artery branches in patients with vessels that cannot be easily catheterized with 5 French PE catheters.

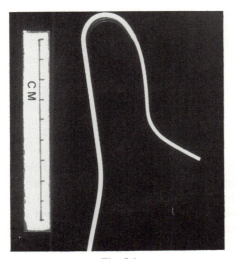
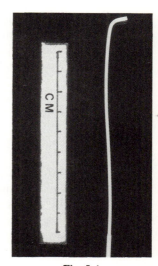

Fig. 5.3   Fig. 5.4

Fig. 5.3 Simmons 'Sidewinder' catheter. Note that the terminal 8 cm tapers abruptly from 7 French to 5 French.

Fig. 5.4 Berenstein 'Hockey Stick' catheter. The terminal 10 cm is tapered to 5 French.

Contrast media

The factors governing the effect of contrast media on the central nervous system have been extensively reviewed (Sage 1983). Side effects are directly related to osmolarity (Grainger 1982), so non-ionic water soluble contrast media (Iopamidol, Iohexol) are ideal. Sodium ioxoglate (Hexabrix), a low osmolarity ionic dimer, is cheaper, but produces more nausea and vomiting than the non-ionic contrast media. An even cheaper acceptable alternative is a contrast medium with a methylglucamine cation, such as Conray 60% (methylglucamine iothalomate), or Angiografin 65% (methylglucamine amidotrizoate), particularly when used in diluted form for intra-arterial DSA. Conventional arch studies require denser contrast media, such as iopamidol 370 mg iodine/100 ml, iohexol 370 mg iodine/100 ml, ioxoglate 300 mg iodine/ml, iothalamate 420 mg iodine/ml, or diatrizoate 370 mg/ml. The lower osmolarity contrast media are particularly suitable for superselective external carotid branch studies, for which only small volumes are required and pain can be minimized.

Other desirable equipment

1. Mechanical pump for standardized injections.
2. Closed flushing system.
3. Sterile, disposable masks, gowns, gloves and surgical hats.
4. Good quality image intensifier and television chain.
5. 100 mA generator capable of at least 3 films/s with small focal spot, 0.3 mm or less. The small focal spot is mandatory for magnification studies.
6. Puck changer.
7. Rare earth screens.

Guidewires

The basic wire for use in cerebral vessels is a fixed core, teflon coated 'long (10 cm) floppy tip' 0.89 mm (0.035 in) diameter straight wire guide. Teflon coated 'J tip' wire guides should only be used as far as the aortic arch, or, occasionally within the external carotid artery, as slight withdrawal of the J wire guide may elevate an athermatous plaque. A broad J wire may be needed to negotiate particularly tortuous carotid arteries, or to allow catheterization of the right subclavian artery and, subsequently, the right vertebral artery. Other wires of occasional usefulness are movable core straight and J wires and straight and curved variable stiffness guidewires (VSG), the stiffness and curve of which are governed by the amount of pressure applied to the deflector handles.

Patient preparation

As for visceral angiography.

In only exceptional cases should it be necessary to add the risk of general anaesthesia (albeit small) to that of the procedure. Even premedication is unnecessary in the majority of cases, after the procedure has been thoroughly explained to the patient, preferably in the ward on the day preceding the examination. For particularly anxious patients, oral diazepam 5–10 mg should be adequate, together with constant communication during the procedure. For procedures involving considerable pain, such as selective external carotid studies and embolization, opiates for pain, together with anti-cholinergic drugs to prevent potential vaso-vagal reactions are desirable. Morphine 10–20 mg, plus atropine 0.6 mg, or Omnopon 10–20 mg, scopolamine 0.2–0.4 mg may need to be used. Neuroleptanalgesia is a more complicated alternative. The respiratory depressant effect of these drugs renders them contraindicated for intracerebral studies, as the resultant increased partial pressure of carbon dioxide will dilate intracerebral arteries with consequent rapid shunting of diluted contrast medium and elevation of intracranial pressure. If general anaesthesia is used, it is desirable to maintain the partial pressure of carbon dioxide between 30 and 35 mm of mercury.

ANGIOGRAPHIC PROCEDURES

Shaping the catheter

Prior to puncture of the common femoral artery a 5F PE catheter is shaped according to the patient's age and anticipated aortic arch shape (Fig. 5.1). In adolescents and young adults tight curves are necessary. With increasing age the second curve may be made progressively longer to conform to an elongated aortic arch.

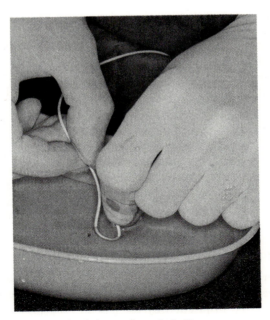

Fig. 5.5 Shaping a 5 French polyethylene catheter in boiling water.

The shape is achieved by holding the catheter in the desired shape with the gloved hands over a jet of steam, or within boiling water for approximately 5 seconds, then transferring it rapidly into cold saline or prep solution (Fig. 5.5).

To avoid kinking a rapid 'prewarming' may be performed. This consists of exposure to the heat source for 1 second only and allows the catheter to be bent to at least half the desired shape without kinking, before again immersing it in the hot water or exposing it to the steam jet.

Catheterization of major arch vessels with 5F catheters

The catheter is introduced into the ascending aorta over a 145 cm 0.89 mm (0.035 in) small J guidewire and the wire removed as soon as possible to prevent loss of catheter shape. In young patients there is a tendency for straight guidewires to pass directly into the left subclavian artery. The catheter may have to be railroaded over the guidewire almost to its tip and the catheter shape used to negotiate the bend between descending aorta and arch. If this fails, the introducing wire should be replaced by a 0.035 broad J guidewire. The broad J wire will always advance into arch and ascending aorta.

If the shape of the arch has been correctly anticipated, the catheter should sit virtually in the arch lumen with its tip facing one of the orifices arising from the superior aspect of the arch (Fig. 5.6b). By gently pulling backwards, the tip should in turn engage the innominate, left common carotid and left subclavian origins. The left common carotid origin may more easily be selected by gently pushing the catheter from the origin of the left subclavian artery. Some gentle twisting of the catheter at the groin may be necessary to encourage the curved portion of the catheter to adopt the upright position in the arch. In particularly ectatic arches it may be necessary to introduce the straight 0.035 guidewire 0.5 to 1 cm beyond the tip of the catheter before the vessel origins can be engaged. A 0.035 straight wire is then gently advanced initially to the level of the fifth cervical vertebra 1–2 cm proximal to the expected level of the carotid bifurcation (Fig. 5.6c). Holding the wire firmly with the right hand to prevent it passing more distally, the catheter is then gently railroaded over the guidewire into the distal common carotid artery (Fig. 5.6d).

At no stage in adults should the 5F catheters be advanced without the flexible end of the guidewire extending beyond the catheter tip.

Techniques for particularly tortuous arteries

In patients with tortuous arteries, it may be necessary to pass the guidewire up to the level of C1 and to extend and rotate the patient's head to the opposite side. Deep inspiration by the patient further straightens the neck vessels, while a deliberate cough by the patient may be the final mechanism

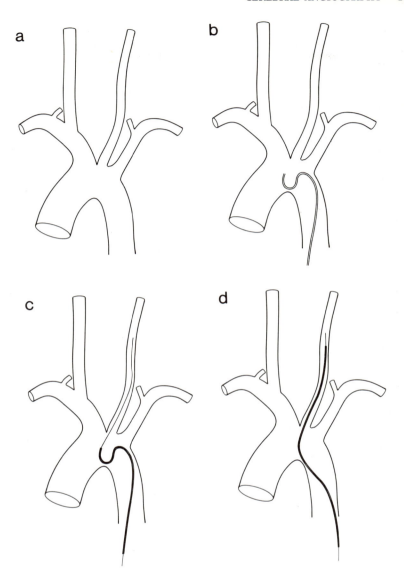

Fig. 5.6 Selective catheterization of the left common carotid artery with a 5 French polyethylene catheter. (a) Normal 'young' aortic arch. (b) Catheter placed in arch with tip facing left common carotid orifice. (c) 0.035 in (0.89 mm) straight guidewire advanced through catheter to the level of the fifth cervical vertebra. (d) Catheter advanced ('railroaded') over guidewire into the left common carotid artery.

of persuading a guide to negotiate a difficult curve. At no stage should manipulation be hurried. Gentle but firm pressure upon the guide and catheter will achieve far more success and safety than impatient, frenzied efforts to pass difficult curves. Pushing only intermittently, the pulsations of the artery alone will on occasions advance catheter or wire past seemingly impossible curves. A broad 'J' wire may be necessary on some occasions to negotiate particularly tortuous vessels. Its increased rigidity means that it does not have to be passed as far distally before supporting the passage of a catheter over it. A VSG straight wire may achieve the same result (Willson 1980). Passed into the carotid or vertebral vessel in its non-rigid floppy state, it can then be rendered sufficiently rigid to support the passage of a catheter over it.

Another described method of negotiating difficult arteries is manual compression of the carotid vessel containing the guidewire by an assistant, which 'anchors' the wire allowing passage of the catheter over it (Chakera & Hartley 1982).

The preformed shape of the Mani PE 5 French catheter (Fig. 5.2) seems particularly useful for engaging the origins of left common carotid arteries in patients with elongated arches and common origins of innominate and left common carotid arteries. Actually pushing the Mani slightly further around the arch of a patient with common origins often induces the tip to point in the direction of the left common carotid artery, allowing a straight guidewire to be directed into the left common carotid artery (Fig. 5.7).

With experience the angiographer will quickly be able to assess the likelihood of success with the 5F PE catheter. Such an assessment should be possible within 10 minutes of beginning the catheterization. The 5F PE

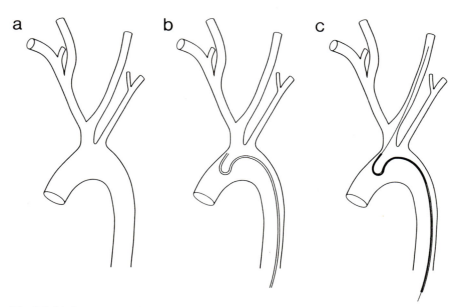

Fig. 5.7 (a) Common origin of innominate and left common carotid arteries. (b) 5 French polyethylene 'Mani' catheter pushed past common origin. (c) 0.035 in (0.89 mm) straight guidewire directed into left common carotid artery.

catheter should then be exchanged either for a Simmons 'Sidewinder III' (Fig. 5.3) or for a Berenstein 'Hockey Stick' catheter (Fig. 5.4).

Technique of catheterization with the 'Sidewinder' catheter

The Simmons 'Sidewinder III' is the catheter of choice for most elongated ectatic arches (Simmons et al 1973). Particularly ectatic arches may require the larger dimensions of a Simmons IV catheter.

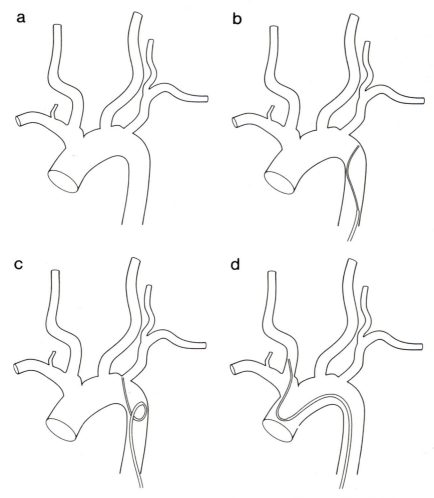

Fig. 5.8 Selective right common carotid catherization with the Simmons 'Sidewinder' catheter. (a) Elongated, 'old' aortic arch. (b) Rotational torque applied as the catheter is advanced in the proximal descending aorta. (c) Acutely angled loop obtained. Rotational torque continued as catheter is further advanced. (d) Catheter acquires its original shape. Required arterial orifice selected by withdrawing catheter.

The 'Sidewinder' catheter is introduced into the proximal segment of the descending aorta over a guidewire and the guidewire is removed. Several methods have been described for reforming the 'Sidewinder' loop. The following simple method works in almost 100% of cases (Fig. 5.8a). The catheter is slowly advanced while at the same time applying a vigorous rotational torque to the catheter just proximal to its entry into the groin (Fig. 5.8b). The rotational motion may be in either direction as long as it is maintained in that single direction. As the catheter traverses the arch it will gradually become more and more acutely angled as it rotates (Fig. 5.8c). By the time it has reached the ascending aorta it will have reassumed its original shape. The catheter is then advanced further into the femoral artery, without any rotational element until its tip is beyond the origin of the required vessel. It is then withdrawn with catheter tip facing superiorly to engage the vessel origin (Fig. 5.8d). Withdrawal is then continued to advance the catheter tip more distally into the required artery.

To remove the catheter from the artery with catheter shape maintained the opposite sequence of movements is performed. The catheter is advanced into the femoral artery at the groin, resulting in withdrawal of the catheter tip from the vessel in the neck. To transfer the catheter from the right to left carotid artery and left carotid to left subclavian artery the catheter is rotated slightly to prevent re-engagement of the catheter tip in the innominate artery and withdrawn at the groin. Once past the innominate origin the catheter is rotated slightly in the reverse direction to re-establish the superiorly directed orientation of the catheter tip and the left common carotid origin is engaged. To pass from the left common carotid to the right innominate artery the catheter is merely advanced at the groin. This action disengages the catheter from the left common carotid origin. Further advancement will result in engagement of the innominate origin.

Technique of catheterization with Berenstein catheter

Because the bulk of both the Berenstein and the Simmons catheters is 7F and more rigid than the 5F cerebral catheters, torque control at the groin is improved dramatically. As with the Simmons catheter most of the users of the Berenstein catheter advocate its use without a guidewire. Its torque control certainly allows it to be directly advanced into the major vessels arising from the arch without a guidewire once it has engaged their origins. If it is intended to pass it selectively into either internal carotid or external carotid artery, the use of a guidewire to facilitate its atraumatic passage through the carotid bifurcation is recommended.

Technique of direct puncture of the common carotid artery

With the patient's head in a neutral or slightly extended position the common carotid artery is palpated at a point in the neck as low as possible, medial to the sternocleidomastoid muscle. The skin is stretched gently towards the head and local anaesthetic (1% xylocaine) is very carefully infiltrated, with frequent syringe plunger withdrawals to prevent any inadvertent injection of local anaesthetic directly into the common carotid artery. A small scalpel blade nick is applied and an 18 gauge disposable, short bevelled arterial needle is introduced through the nick with the skin still stretched towards the cranium. One or more of the fingers of the left hand, usually the index and middle fingers, are used to palpate the artery distal to the needle and the right hand carefully advances the needle, which is held at a steeper angle than that used for femoral artery puncture e.g. 70–80° to the skin surface (Fig. 5.9).

The point of the needle will transmit the arterial pulsation to the right hand when in contact with the artery. When maximum pulsation is transmitted from the needle to the right hand and gentle pressure with the needle leads to a decrease in the pressure of pulsation in the artery under the left finger, the needle is in contact with the centre of the artery. A rapid, firm movement with the right hand will usually result in both walls being transfixed by the needle. The left hand is removed and the needle gently withdrawn. When it is withdrawn from the posterior wall, the reflex recoil of the stretched skin will signal the entry of the needle into the arterial lumen by a palpable click and a reorientation of the needle, which will point more acutely in a cranial direction. Pulsatile blood is immediately received

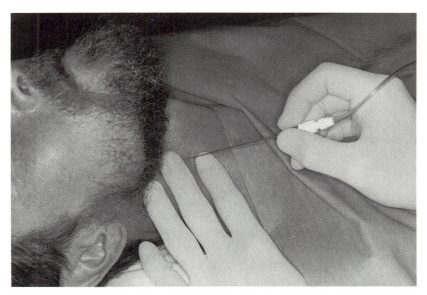

Fig. 5.9 Direct carotid puncture. With index finger and forefinger palpating the common carotid artery medial to the sternomastoid muscle, skin is stretched towards cranium before needle is advanced.

in the syringe. Heparinized saline at minute intervals should be flushed through the syringe to prevent clotting of the needle and tubing. No further manipulation of the needle should be needed. A rapid test injection of 1–2 ml of contrast medium should be performed under fluoroscopy to ensure that the tip of the needle is not deep to the intima, as relatively free backflow of pulsatile blood can still take place if most of the bevel of the needle is within the lumen. Contrast medium injection by hand or machine can now be performed, at the rates and volumes specified below.

Transaxillary carotid arteriography

Alternative carotid approaches, such as transbrachial and transaxillary using the Simmons III catheter have been described (Kerber et al 1975), but should not be necessary in the era of digital subtraction angiography. Once practised, direct carotid puncture is far faster and safer than the transaxillary approach.

Selective catheterization

Internal and external carotid arteries

Before selectively catheterizing the internal or external carotid artery the bifurcation in the neck should be visualized to ensure that the internal carotid artery is not stenosed and to determine the exact relationship of the internal and external carotid artery origins. For angiographic laboratories with only vertical fluoroscopic facilities, this is best achieved by rotating the head of the patient as far as possible away from the side being studied and injecting 1–2 ml of contrast medium forcefully by hand. Horizontal beam screening facilities are ideal for the purpose. As the internal carotid artery usually passes postero-laterally from the bifurcation and the external carotid artery passes antero-medially, torque should be applied at the groin to cause the tip of the catheter immediately proximal to the bifurcation to point towards the desired vessel. The straight 0.035 wire should then be advanced well into the appropriate vessel and the catheter railroaded over the guide. In the external carotid artery, there may be a tendency for the guidewire to enter one of the more proximal branches, such as superior thyroid or facial artery. Gentle torque in the groin will usually change the direction of the catheter to allow passage of the guide past the branch orifices. If not, the situation constitutes probably the one indication for the use of the tight J 0.035 guide within the cerebral vessels, as its J tip will usually allow the guide to pass up the main stem of the external carotid artery.

If difficulty is encountered in pointing the catheter in the common carotid towards the desired vessel, it is helpful to know that in most patients a straight guidewire passed through the common carotid artery will enter the internal carotid artery and a broad J guidewire will enter the external carotid artery.

In both the internal carotid artery and external carotid artery the catheter tip should be positioned at least 3–4 cm from the bifurcation to prevent reflux of contrast media, or even dislodgement of the catheter from its selected position by the pressure of the injection. If vertical fluoroscopy has been used, it is judicious to check the position of the catheter after the head has been rotated back to the neutral position, as this movement alone may dislodge the catheter, or, conversely, cause it to engage superselectively with an unwanted external carotid branch.

External carotid artery branches

Deliberate superselective external carotid arterylography is most easily performed with horizontal beam fluoroscopy. If difficulty is still encountered in identifying the individual branches, a short lateral neck angiographic series should precede further attempts at catheterization. A knowledge of the normal origins of each branch is essential. Using the curves in the terminal segment of the catheter to 'point' towards the required branch, its orifice can usually be engaged without the use of a guidewire. Only in the external carotid artery should the catheter be advanced without a guidewire projecting from the end. Excessive manipulation may induce spasm in the external carotid artery, for which the only known treatment is to cease manipulation in that vessel for 20 minutes or more.

Vertebral artery

Left vertebral artery. Unless there is a specific need for a right vertebral artery study, left vertebral artery catheterization should be attempted first. The left vertebral artery is either the dominant vessel, or is at least equal in size to the right vertebral artery in 70% of patients. This is fortunate, as it is generally the easier of the two to catheterize, a fact which inexperienced angiographers passing a straight guidewire retrogradely too far up the descending aorta will quickly come to realize. Ideally, the catheter tip should first be positioned in the subclavian origin and a test injection of 1–2 ml of contrast medium made to confirm that a left vertebral artery is indeed present (4% of left vertebral arteries arise directly from the arch between the left common carotid and left subclavian origins) and to establish its point of origin. In addition, it will be apparent in most cases whether the left vertebral artery is of sufficient size to catheterize safely. If not, right vertebral artery catheterization should be attempted first.

As the left vertebral artery arises from the medial aspect of the ascending portion of the left subclavian artery in most cases, it will usually be necessary to turn the tip of the catheter so that it, too, faces medially before advancing the 0.035 straight guidewire. If the vertebral origin is tortuous, a movable core guidewire may negotiate the curves with the core retracted.

The catheter can then be advanced over the guide after the core has been replaced. Neither the wire nor the catheter tip should be advanced beyond the level of C3, so as to avoid damage to the vessel as it passes acutely laterally from the transverse foramen of C3 to that of C2. If any resistance to forward movement is encountered, no attempt should be made to advance the catheter past the proximal segment of the artery. If guide and catheter pass easily, the tip can be carefully positioned as high as the C3–C4 disc. A careful test injection of 1/2 to 1 ml is necessary to assess the size of the vertebral artery and the rate at which contrast medium disappears. If there is any undue delay in the rate of disappearance of the contrast medium this indicates that the catheter at some point is nearly occluding the lumen and it should be immediately withdrawn.

Right vertebral artery. The catheter tip is placed in the innominate origin. In some patients, it may be possible to induce a straight 0.035 guidewire to enter the subclavian rather than the right common carotid artery by quickly rotating the catheter in a clockwise direction before passing the guidewire. More commonly it is necessary to pass a broad J 0.035 guidewire into the innominate origin. It will preferentially pass into the subclavian artery and even on occasions, directly into the right vertebral artery. After removal of the guidewire the catheter is gently withdrawn, rotating if necessary to persuade the terminal tip to point towards the superior aspect of the subclavian artery and engage the right vertebral artery origin. A straight 0.035 guidewire is then advanced into the right vertebral artery and the catheter railroaded over the guidewire. The placement of catheter tip and assessment of right vertebral artery size are performed in the same manner as on the left.

Alternative approaches to vertebral angiography

If these methods are unsuccessful or selective catheterization is vital, a transaxillary or transbrachial approach, using a catheter with its terminal tip turned through 90°, will usually be successful. Special catheter shapes have been described for difficult vertebral arteries (Guinto 1982). With the advent of DSA it should be unnecessary to perform direct vertebral puncture, a procedure with an unacceptably high degree of risk in inexperienced hands. The injection of contrast medium into the subclavian artery with or without an inflated sphygmanometer cuff applied to the upper arm will allow sufficient contrast medium to enter the vertebral artery for a satisfactory DSA.

Cerebral angiography–radiographic techniques

The radiographic techniques used should pragmatically vary with the indication for the examination to minimize radiation exposure and cost. For the evaluation of the cerebral vessels of a patient who has had a subarachnoid haemorrhage it is essential to obtain detailed images of the arterial phase from at least 3 separate projections. The capillary and venous phases need not be recorded in such detail.

For the evaluation of transient ischaemic attacks, views of the internal carotid artery origins, carotid siphon and major internal carotid artery branches are essential. Capillary and venous phases must still be recorded to exclude the occasional tumour or subdural haemorrhage which may clinically simulate a transient ischaemic attack.

For the evaluation of a subtle, non-diagnostic lesion on CT, or for the investigation of suspected arteritis, a long detailed study of the dynamics of cerebral blood flow using magnification and a small focal spot are required.

The delineation of the arterial feeders to an arteriovenous malformation requires a rapid series of films in the arterial phase — at least 3/s.

Contrast medium quantities and rates also vary with the clinical indication. While for most internal carotid artery selective studies 8 ml of contrast medium at 5 ml/s is adequate, for the evaluation of a large, high flow fistula 12 ml at 10 ml/s may be needed.

25 × 30 cm and 35 × 35 cm Puck changers are the standard changers used for cerebral angiography. The 35 × 35 cm changer may be used for the lateral projection with a small focal spot, an air gap between patient and changer, no grid and a piece of lead rubber cut in the shape of a keyhole applied to the film changer (Fig. 5.10). It is then possible to demonstrate the intracerebral and neck circulation in a single angiographic series (Fig. 5.11), thus halving the number of contrast medium injections.

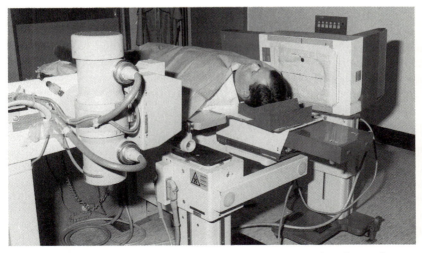

Fig. 5.10 Keyhole shaped lead rubber is applied to the lateral Puck film changer for 'vascular' studies.

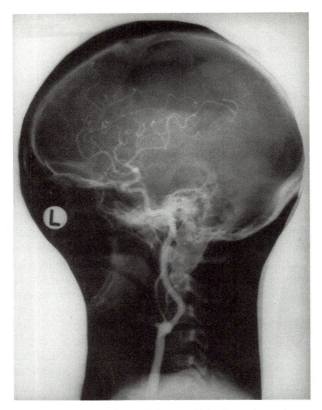

Fig. 5.11 Both intracerebral circulation and the carotid in the neck are demonstrated with one angiographic sequence.

All contrast medium injections are ideally performed with the aid of a mechanical pump to standardize injection rates. Injection rates and volume are individually checked by the radiologist, nurse and radiographer for each injection. A mask radiograph is exposed immediately before contrast medium injection to allow analogue subtraction when required.

Digital subtraction angiography (DSA)

The technique for both intravenous and intra-arterial DSA of the cerebral circulation is covered in the general angiography section. For intra-arterial studies the general principle is that the same volume of contrast medium is injected, diluted by at least 50% with sterile water.

Complications of cerebral angiography

Procedural complications elsewhere in the body, such as peripheral emboliz-ation or intimal dissection, may have a negligible result compared with the catastrophic effect of the same complications in the arteries supplying the central nervous system.

The most serious complication is death, which has an incidence of less than 0.1% (Olivecrona 1977, Earnest et al 1983). Permanent neurological deficits occur in 0.63 to 0.9% of cases. They are due largely to iatrogenic emboli, much less often to contrast medium toxicity. The vertebral arteries are particularly susceptible to contrast medium toxicity, probably as a function of the rate of flow through the vertebrobasilar system and, hence, the length of time the contrast medium is in contact with the vessel intima. Certainly, such complications are more common and severe in the presence of spasm and/or vertebrobasilar stenosis.

Severe complications are more common in patients being investigated for symptomatic cerebrovascular disease (Faught et al 1979, Earnest et al 1983). They are more common when large bore, relatively rigid catheters are used, rather than smaller (5F), softer PE catheters (Kerber et al 1978, Mani et al 1978). Other factors associated with increased risk of neurological deficit include old age, increased serum creatinine and the use of more than one catheter.

Intimal dissection is not nearly as common with catheter angiography as it was with direct carotid and vertebral puncture. Injection of contrast medium into the subarachnoid space is a complication only of direct vertebral artery puncture. Tracheal obstruction rarely results from direct carotid artery punctures, particularly bilateral. Other minor non-neurological complications, including groin haematoma, contrast medium extravasation, transient hypertension, allergic reactions, occur more often (8.5%), but have no permanent sequelae (Earnest et al 1983).

Reduction of complications

The importance of meticulous attention to technical detail cannot be emphasized enough. Specifically, the following recommendations must be adhered to:

1. Rigidly aseptic technique.
2. Guidewires should not be allowed to remain in any catheter for more than 1 minute. Scrupulous catheter toilet after guidewire removal is mandatory.
3. Catheters and guidewires should be used only once.
4. The expertise of angiographic and radiographic staff, as well as nurse assistants, must be developed rapidly to enable minimum operational time.
5. The procedure should be immediately abandoned if the patient develops a neurological deficit.
6. Contrast medium should be regarded as a potentially dangerous neurotoxin. The quantity of contrast medium used must be kept to the minimum amount possible, particularly in the vertebral arteries, into

which an absolute maximum of 5 injections of contrast medium for conventional studies should be performed.

7. Floppy tipped guidewires should always be protruding through the end of any 5F catheter before advance in the common carotid or internal carotid arteries is attempted.

8. Alternative techniques, such as intra-arterial and intravenous DSA, should be used whenever practicable to minimize contrast medium dose.

9. The first angiographic series performed upon patients with subarachnoid haemorrhage, preferably in the AP projection, should be screened for spasm before proceeding to further contrast medium injections. If spasm is severe, the rest of the examination should be postponed for at least 5 days. It should be noted that the clinical state of the patient does not always correlate with the degree of spasm.

10. If on screening the carotid bifurcation it appears to be severely stenosed or occluded, a lateral angiographic series only should be performed before proceeding further. If the stenosis is confirmed to be severe or the vessel occluded, the catheter should be removed from the vessel immediately and the other carotid catheterized.

SPINAL ANGIOGRAPHY

Indications

1. Myelographic diagnosis of arteriovenous malformation.
2. Suspected cord haemangioblastoma.
3. Subarachnoid haemorrhage with strong clinical indication of spinal origin.
4. Investigation of intramedullary haemorrhage in spinal cord.

Preparation

As for visceral angiography. Local anaesthetic only is required in adults, general anaesthesia in children. In view of the likely length of the procedure and to reduce the likelihood of myoclonus, premedication with 10 mg of oral diazepam 20 minutes before the procedure is advisable. Prior to the application of sterile drapes several opaque numbers should be attached to the patient's back, immediately lateral to the vertebral bodies over the corresponding ribs. These are essential for identification of the level of any intercostal artery catheterized during the procedure. The level may then be easily checked fluoroscopically.

Methods

Cervical spinal angiography requires selective catheterization of both vertebral arteries, both thyrocervical trunks and both costocervical trunks, as anterior radiculo-medullary arteries may arise from vertebral, ascending cervical or deep cervical arteries.

Thoraco-lumbar spinal angiography requires selective catheterization of all the intercostal arteries from T4 to T12, all the lumbar arteries and, possibly, the presacral branches of the internal iliac arteries. Even after identification of feeding vessels to an angioma, it is essential to identify the arteria radicularis magna (artery of Adamkiewicz) prior to surgery, as it constitutes almost the entire supply to the anterior spinal artery in the thoraco-lumbar portion of the spinal cord.

Materials

Catheters

For cervical spinal angiography, 5F PE cerebral catheters may be used. In younger patients a simple 60° angle on the terminal centimeter of the catheter is all that is required. For elderly patients the cerebral shapes will be necessary (Fig. 5.1). Should extra torque control be necessary, the Berenstein 'Hockey Stick' catheter (Fig. 5.4) may be used. 4F PE catheters with 60° angulation on the terminal 1 cm are suitable for use in young children.

For thoraco-lumbar spinal angiography, preferred catheters are the Hilal spinal catheter, the Cobra 2 (Fig. 5.12), or the Simmons 'Sidewinder III' cerebral catheter (Fig. 5.3). The Michaelson catheter, with its distinctive

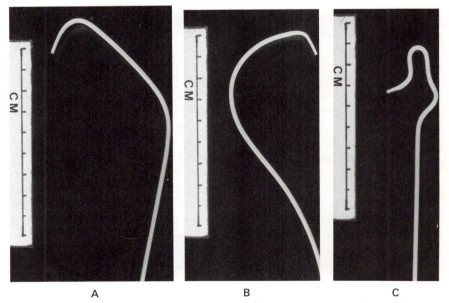

A   B   C

Fig. 5.12 Catheters for use in spinal angiography. (A) Hilal spinal catheter. (B) Cobra 2. (C) Michaelson.

shepherd's crook shape, has a more limited use in particularly ectatic aortas (Fig. 5.12).

Contrast media

Contrast media with organic cations or non-ionic contrast media are preferred, as sodium cations are toxic to neural tissue. Methylglucamine iothalamate is the contrast medium of choice, if the expense of the non-ionic contrast media precludes their exclusive use. However, non-ionic contrast media may be used in larger volumes when a more detailed study of specific feeding vessels is required. If a water soluble contrast medium is to be used it should be made up to a concentration of at least 280 mg of iodine/ml. The concentration of contrast medium may be halved when intra-arterial DSA is available.

Technique

Conventional midstream aortograms are of little use in detecting abnormal feeders and add intolerably to what is in many cases an already large contrast medium load. However, using intra-arterial DSA, a midstream aortogram may indicate the larger feeders to the racemose type of arteriovenous malformation seen in childhood. The adult type of arteriovenous malformation usually has only one or two feeding vessels, which may still require selective catheterization for their identification.

Cervical spinal angiography. Selective vertebral artery studies are obtained, as described in the section on cerebral angiography. To catheterize thyrocervical and costocervical trunks a broad J wire is passed through the catheter stationed in left subclavian or innominate artery origins. It will usually pass distally into the subclavian artery. The catheter is railroaded over the wire into the distal subclavian and the wire removed. As the catheter is withdrawn, torque is applied to the catheter in the groin to induce its distal tip to point superiorly and in turn engage the origins of costocervical trunk, thyrocervical trunk and vertebral artery. On only very rare occasions should a subclavian or brachial arterial approach be necessary. Selective catheterization via these routes can be achieved using a catheter with a simple 60° angulation in its terminal 1 cm.

Thoraco-lumbar spinal angiography. In the younger patient both left and right intercostal arteries project symmetrically postero-laterally from the aorta. Once one intercostal artery has been located, merely passing the catheter straight along the aorta without rotating the catheter will enable rapid catheterization of all the ipsilateral intercostal vessels. The contralateral vessels can be catheterized in the same manner. With aging, the aorta tends to elongate and rotate to the left. Consequently both left and right intercostal arteries tend to project from the right side of the aorta, as seen with vertical fluoroscopy in the supine patient. Catheter changes may be necessary or a loop may have to be produced in the Cobra catheter for lower lumbar artery catheterization (see section on 'Selective abdominal angiography', p. 87). Test injections of contrast medium should be of small volume (0.5–1 ml) to minimize both contrast medium total load and individual vessel contrast medium load.

The contralateral presacral artery is usually readily catheterizable with the Cobra catheter and in many cases so is the ipsilateral presacral artery, using the technique described to obtain a recurved tip in Chapter 4. Occasionally, it will be necessary to enter the contralateral femoral artery to catheterize the ipsilateral presacral artery.

Radiographic technique

Initially, only an AP projection is utilised. A lateral projection will give further information, when an abnormal feeder has been isolated in the AP projection. Magnification, using at least a 0.3 mm focal spot, is extremely helpful, when used in conjunction with analogue subtraction. Intra-arterial DSA is of particular value, when compared with conventional magnification studies, despite slightly decreased spatial resolution. It is more rapid, allows a smaller total contrast medium dose and is more comfortable for the patient.

Film sequences

Cervical Spinal Angiography
(a) Vertebral artemes 1 film/s for 7 s. 8 ml of contrast medium may be injected at a rate of 5 ml/s.
(b) Thyrocervical and costocervical trunks: 1 film every 2 s for 8 s 4 ml of contrast medium may be injected at a rate of 2 ml/s.

Thoraco-lumbar spinal angiography
(a) Intercostal and lumbar arteries: 1 film every 2 s for 8 s. 3–4 ml of contrast medium may be injected at a maximum rate of 2 ml/s. When a major feeding vessel is discovered it may be necessary to use a large bolus of non-ionic contrast medium, such as 8 ml of non-ionic water soluble contrast medium in which the iodine concentration is 280–300 mg iodine/ml. 8 ml may be injected at a rate of 3 ml/s while radiographs are exposed at 1 second intervals for a total of 8 s. If a very slow flowing vascular malformation is revealed, the film sequence may have to be extended. In every case, a mask radiograph is exposed before contrast medium injection.

LUMBAR VENOGRAPHY

Indication

In the past this study constituted the method of choice for evaluation of the lumbosacral nerve roots when the epidural space was abnormally wide, or myelography was contraindicated. It has been largely superseded by lumbar CT.

Technique

Using a 5F PE catheter with a simple 60° bend in its terminal 1 cm, the ascending lumbar vein may be catheterized via a left femoral vein approach. A second catheter may be introduced into the contralateral lateral sacral vein by catheterizing the contralateral internal iliac vein and applying torque to induce the tip of the catheter to face medially. Abdominal compression should be applied, the patient made to perform the Valsalva manoeuvre and 30 ml of standard angiographic contrast medium can be injected simultaneously at a rate of 8 ml/s. AP magnification radiographs of the lumbar spine are obtained at the rate of 1/s for 10 s. Subtraction is again helpful. All radicular veins and veins of the anterior internal vertebral venous plexus should be opacified on both sides of the affected level. This is necessary to confirm satisfactory filling of all significant veins. If there is any doubt the study should be repeated with the catheter tips in slightly different positions, as there is some evidence that slight changes in position can lead to artefact or non-filling of radicular veins.

Complication

Apart from the occasional rupture of an injected vein morbidity is low, virtually that of the contrast medium alone.

JUGULAR VENOGRAPHY

Indications

1. Assessment of degree of invasion of jugular vein by glomus tumours.
2. Confirmation of diagnosis of sigmoid or lateral sinus thrombosis.
3. Confirmation of congenitally large jugular bulb seen on skull radiographs as an apparent erosion.
4. Rarely, as a conduit to the inferior petrosal and cavernous sinuses for the percutaneous obliteration of carotico-cavernous fistulae.

Techniques

1. Indirect. The venous phase of a conventional internal carotid angiogram will usually include adequate views of the internal jugular vein, particularly if enhanced by magnification and subtraction. The venous phase of intravenous DSA will show all sinuses simultaneously.

2. Direct. Transfemoral jugular venography is simply performed via either common femoral vein in the groin. Puncture technique is as described previously. A 5F PE catheter with a simple 60° angulation of the terminal 1 cm is introduced over a 0.89 mm tight J guidewire. The guidewire will usually pass from inferior vena cava through the right atrium into the superior vena cava. Occasionally, the catheter will have to be rail-roaded as far as the tip of the guidewire, thus inducing a bend which can be used for directing the guide into the superior vena cava. The shape is again used to catheterize the appropriate innominate and internal jugular veins. The catheter tip should be positioned 1 to 2 cm below the jugular bulb. 15 ml of 60% contrast medium is then injected at the rate of 10 ml/s while radiographs are exposed at the rate of 2/s for 5 s in an AP projection. The series can then be repeated in the lateral projection and, if the anatomy is still not clearly demonstrated, in the submento-vertical projection.

Interior petrosal sinus selective catheterization. The interior petrosal sinuses drain into the internal jugular veins approximately 1 cm inferior to the dome of the jugular bulb. Therefore, after catheterization of the internal jugular vein, the catheter tip should be directed antero-medially approximately 1 cm below the apex of the jugular bulk to engage the interior petrosal sinus.

Complications

These are largely limited to those of the contrast medium itself. The patient may complain of a buzzing sound in the ear. In the rare situation in which friable clot may be present, some degree of pulmonary embolization may result, usually without symptoms.

Cavernous sinus thrombosis is a rare complication of inferior petrosal sinus selective catheterization.

ORBITAL VENOGRAPHY

Orbital venography has been almost entirely replaced by orbital CT. Its indications are now very limited.

Indications

1. Delineation of the anatomy of orbital varices (the diagnosis is a clinical one) prior to surgery.
2. Confirmation of diagnosis of Tolosa–Hunt syndrome.

Techniques

The most appropriate method is direct cannulation of a frontal vein on the forehead. A 19 gauge scalp vein needle can be used after the venous pressure has been elevated by positioning the patient with head dependent and placing rubber bands around neck and upper forehead. These should

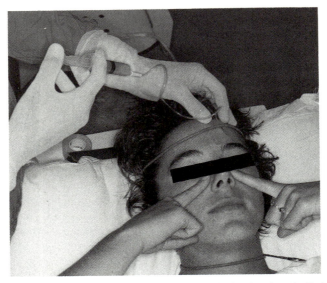

Fig. 5.13 Orbital phlebography. Tourniquets applied to forehead and neck. Patient compresses anterior facial veins.

be of sufficient tension to occlude venous flow while preserving arterial flow. Compression pads, or the patient's own fingers, should be used to compress the facial veins over the maxillae (Fig. 5.13).

10 ml of 60% contrast medium is injected as fast as is practicable without rupturing the veins. The maximum allowable flow rate is carefully assessed by gently injecting normal saline. The standard projection is AP with tube angled cranially 20° to project the orbits above the petrous bones. The submento-vertical projection delineates the cavernous sinuses. The lateral view is of limited value, because of the superimposition of both orbital venous networks. Films are exposed at a rate of 1/s for 8 films.

Complications

Venous rupture and chemically induced cellulitis at the site of rupture is the most common complication. Careful puncture and saline test injections help reduce the incidence of this complication.

MYELOGRAPHY

The indications for myelography have been reduced with the advent of spinal CT and CT assisted myelography and will be reduced even further when magnetic resonance imagers are widely available. The almost complete replacement of oily contrast media by water soluble contrast media has resulted in the need for an even more obsessive technical approach, if high quality studies are to be consistently produced.

Indications

Water soluble contrast media

1. Sciatica syndrome, with normal or equivocal CT.
2. Cervical radicular pain.
3. Suspected spinal tumour (intramedullary, extramedullary and extradural) if MRI is not available.
4. Suspected spinal arteriovenous malformation.
5. Investigation of residual or recurrent symptoms and signs after laminectomy, if CT is equivocal.

Oily contrast media

6. Previous adverse reaction to water soluble contrast media.

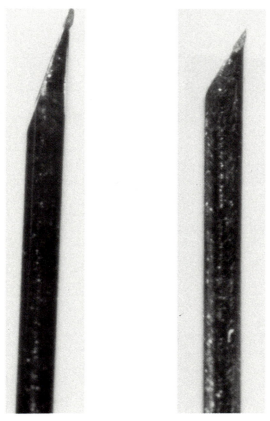

Fig. 5.14 Magnified view of tips of 22 gauge disposable lumbar puncture needles, conventional on left and short bevel on right.

Equipment

Twenty-two gauge, short bevelled disposable lumbar puncture needles can be used for both lumbar and cervical punctures for the introduction of water soluble contrast media (Fig. 5.14). More appropriate for use with the more viscous oily contrast media (Fig. 5.15) are 18 gauge disposable lumbar puncture needles with insertable blunt ended cannulae for contrast medium withdrawal.

Plastic tubing, at least 30 cm long, enables contrast media to be injected under screening control. Local anaesthetic, in the form of 1% or 2% xylocaine, should be used for puncture with 19 or 20 gauge needles and for 22 gauge needles in inexperienced hands. Aqueous chlorhexidine solution, swabs, 20 ml disposable plastic syringes, drawing up needles and disposable 23 or 25 gauge needles for local anaesthetic and sterile drapes constitute the basic necessities, other than the contrast medium itself. A tilt table,

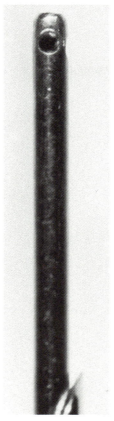

Fig. 5.15 Blunt ended cannula inserted through 18 gauge lumbar puncture needle to allow atraumatic withdrawal of oily contrast medium.

preferably tilting 90° in at least one direction, biplane screening facilities, generators capable of low KVP exposures in 70 KVP range and Iontomat exposure control are ideal.

Contrast media

Water soluble non-ionic

1. Iohexol
2. Iopamidol
3. Metrizamide
   Dosages. Dose is dependent on the indication and the body habitus.
   Lumbar myelography. 10–13 ml in concentrations of iodine 200 to 220 mg/ml.
   Thoracic myelography. 10–13 ml in concentrations of iodine 240 to 300 mg/ml (maximum 3 g of iodine).
   Cervical myelography. 5–10 ml in concentration of iodine 300 mg/ml (maximum 3 g of iodine).

Oily contrast media

1. Iophendylate (Myodil, Pantopaque).
   Dosages
   Lumbar myelography: 6–12 ml
   Thoracic myelography: 15–24 ml
   Cervical myelography: 12–18 ml
   Whole of spine: 24 ml
   Diagnosis of block: 3–6 ml

Air

There is no longer any reasonable indication for air myelography.

Patient preparation

1. Pre-procedure discussion with the patient, preferably on the day preceeding the investigation, is the best method of calming the patient's fears and assessing the need for medication.
2. All phenothiazine and tricyclic anti-depressant therapy should be discontinued 48 hours prior to the examination.
3. Diazepam 10 mg orally should be given 1 hour prior to the examination only if the patient is markedly anxious.
4. Hydration should be continued right up until the examination, although solid food should be discontinued 4 hours prior to examination.

Technique

Water soluble myelography

The basis of water soluble myelography technique is the elimination of any unnecessary patient movement or posturing. Because the contrast medium is heavier than water and CSF, it will form a layer in the dependent part of the subarachnoid space, providing it is not agitated. Because of its complete water miscibility, any movement of the patient will lead to some dissemination of the contrast medium, with resultant decreased contrast medium density. Hence, the most desirable patient positioning for needle puncture is prone for both lumbar and cervical myelography, performed via either a lateral cervical or lumbar approach.

Lumbar myelography

Lumbar puncture should be midline with the patient prone. If a midline puncture proves impossible, the bevel of the needle may be used to deliberately bend the puncture needle, allowing successful lateral puncture (Fig. 5.16).

If for any reason the prone position is not possible nor obtainable, a lumbar puncture performed with the patient sitting hunched over pillows,

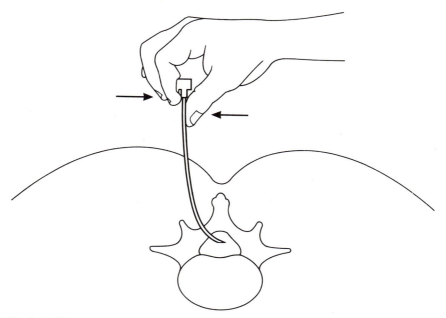

Fig. 5.16 The application of pressure to the needle by thumb and forefinger while it is being advanced results in a curved needle path, allowing a midline entry into the theca from a lateral puncture.

or lying on one side may be used. The dose and concentration of contrast medium used varies with the body habitus of the patient and the capacity of the spinal subarachnoid space. For young, slim patients, concentrations of 200 mg of iodine per ml of contrast medium should be sufficient, while for larger patients, 240 mg of iodine per ml may be necessary. The volume of contrast medium needed for the average study is that necessary to cover the L3–L4 disc space with the patient prone and the table tilted 30° head up. Thus, in severe spinal stenosis 6 ml may prove sufficient, while patients with dural ectasia will require the maximum volume of the larger concentration.

After removal of only sufficient CSF for the required laboratory tests, contrast medium should be slowly injected while screening with the patient 30° head up. Carefully coned AP radiographs on the serial changer and a horizontal beam lateral radiograph should be obtained without moving the patient. Once these have been checked and found to be technically satisfactory an AP oblique study should be performed. 2° of obliquity are recommended, usually 15° and 30°, as the nerve root sheaths in profile are seen best in some patients at 15° and in others at steeper degrees of obliquity. These two obliques should be exposed on one split film and the procedure repeated on a second split film for the opposite oblique studies. Thus, AP, horizontal beam lateral and AP oblique radiographs form the essential part of the study.

Optional views include erect lateral views taken on the serial changer with the patient in flexion and extension and horizontal beam decubitus lateral projections, but these should only be performed after the essential series as they, of necessity, will produce some diffusion of the contrast medium throughout the CSF.

At the completion of the study, contrast medium should be carefully manipulated up to the level of the conus medullaris and AP radiographs of the conus region exposed. This may be difficult in the prone position for patients with a pronounced lumbar lordosis, in which case the patient should be turned supine and contrast medium moved into the thoracic kyphosis, where an above couch AP 43 × 17 cm film of the thoraco-lumbar spine should be exposed. The patient should then reassume the head up position and be returned to the ward. Both in transit and in the ward bed the patient's head should be elevated at least 30° and the position maintained for at least 6 hours.

Cervical myelography

There are 3 potential sites of introduction of water soluble contrast medium in the cervical region. They are:
1. Lateral C1–C2 puncture.
2. Cisternal puncture.
3. Lumbar puncture.

Because water soluble contrast media are diluted by movement, the most appropriate site is that which will require minimal patient movement, e.g. lateral C1–C2 puncture. In addition, it is impossible to prevent some contrast medium introduced via the other two sites from passing into the cranial subarachnoid space in high concentration, even if the patient's head is fully extended.

Lateral C1–C2 puncture. It is strongly recommended that this route be routinely used only if horizontal beam screening facilities are available. The patient is positioned prone with the head in only slight extension (Fig. 5.17). Full extension will produce buckling of the ligamentum flavum and some resultant compromise of the posterior subarachnoid space. After routine cleansing and draping of the neck inferior to the pinna of the ear, a metallic object is applied to the skin and horizontal beam screening is used to determine the exact point of entry for the needle. The required point of entry is within the posterior one-third of the spinal canal between the neural arches of C1 and C2 (Fig. 5.18). Local anaesthetic is used to raise a small bleb in the epidermis. A 22 gauge, short bevelled spinal needle is then advanced horizontally, regularly checking its progress with the horizontal beam fluoroscope. It is usually difficult to feel 'give' of the dura when using this method so the trochar should be withdrawn and the needle slowly turned through 180° when it is felt that the needle is close to the subarachnoid space. Because there is no head of pressure forcing CSF out and the needle gauge is small, the droplets may take several seconds to appear at the end of the needle (Fig. 5.19).

If it is felt that the needle has been advanced to an appropriate depth, vertical beam screening may be employed to check the position of the needle tip in relation to the midline structures. It should be remembered that the needle tip frequently invaginates the theca in front of it up to 1 cm before piercing it (Orrison et al 1983), so it may have to cross the midline slightly, as seen by AP screening, before achieving entry into the subar-

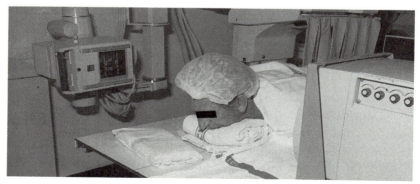

Fig. 5.17 Patient position for lateral C1–C2 puncture. Head only slightly extended. Note horizontal screening apparatus.

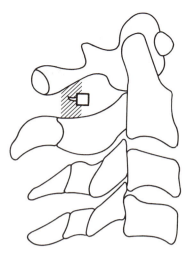

Fig. 5.18 Diagram demonstrating initial needle puncture site in the posterior one-third of the cervical spinal canal between the laminae of C1 and C2.

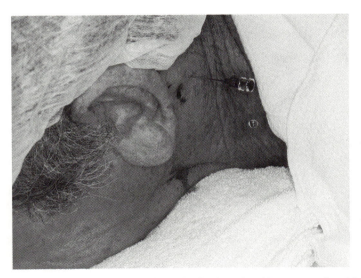

Fig. 5.19 Cerebrospinal fluid drips relatively slowly through a 22 gauge needle with the patient lying prone. Patience is mandatory.

achnoid space. If the first advance is unsuccessful, the needle is angled more anteriorly and the procedure repeated.

After collection of a small specimen of CSF for the required pathology tests, contrast medium is carefully introduced under horizontal beam fluoroscopic control. This point is vital to the success of the whole procedure. A slight tilt of the patient's head too far cranially or caudally can result in almost all the contrast medium being inadvertently tipped into the cranial or lumbar subarachnoid spaces respectively. The contrast medium should pool in the cervical lordosis. A sufficient volume of contrast medium should be used in most cases to extend from clivus to cervico-dorsal junction. The needle is withdrawn.

Still without moving the patient, AP and horizontal beam lateral radiographs are exposed. Only after they have been developed and found to be satisfactory are further radiographs exposed. If the clinical findings indicate a low cervical level, a cervico-dorsal junction horizontal beam lateral is exposed after slowly and passively extending one of the patient's arms cranially to a position parallel to his head. The 30° oblique AP studies are the last prone films performed, as positioning the patient for the oblique projection inevitably results in some dispersion of the contrast medium. If the dorsal subarachnoid space must be opacified to eliminate a foramen magnum lesion and CT is not available to study this region four hours after the myelogram, the patient may be quickly turned supine and an autotomogram performed to expose the sagittal midline plane (Doyle & Tress 1983).

Upon completion of the study the patient should be returned to the ward in the head up position, a position which should be maintained for at least 6 hours, as for lumbar myelography.

Cisternal puncture

Indications for use. The determination of the upper level of a spinal block, when the absence of horizontal beam screening facilities prevents a lateral C1–C2 puncture.

Technique. The patient lies on his side with back towards the radiologist. A firm pillow to prevent any head movement is essential. A telephone book covered by a towel is ideal. The patient's head must be facing directly horizontally for the duration of the procedure.

A small area of hair in the midline of the neck between the tips of the mastoid processes is shaved and the neck sterilized and draped. A small bleb of local anaesthetic is raised in the epidermis at the midline and infiltrated into the dermis. Because the needle must traverse the tough ligamentum nuchae, it is advisable to use a larger bore, more rigid needle. A 20 gauge short bevelled lumbar puncture needle will usually suffice. The needle is introduced in the midline at the level of the mastoid tips and advanced in the direction of the nasion (Fig. 5.20).

The direction and depth should be frequently checked, using the serial changer fluoroscopy unit. The needle should enter the subarachnoid space between the posterior margin of the foramen magnum and the arch of the atlas. The table is tilted feet down some 30° and contrast medium is introduced under fluoroscopic control. After removal of the needle, the patient may be turned prone for conventional AP and lateral radiographs.

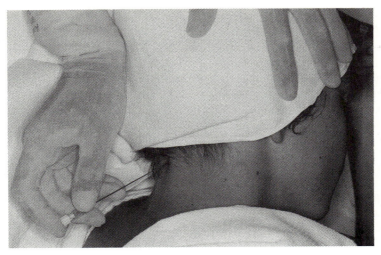

Fig. 5.20 Cisternal puncture. The needle is introduced in the midline between the mastoid processes and angled towards the nasion.

Lumbar puncture

Indications
1. No fluoroscopy facilities available.
2. Foramen magnum lesion suspected.

Technique. The puncture is performed as described above for lumbar myelography. However, the contrast medium is introduced with patient prone, head extended and the table tilted cranially 15 to 20° to facilitate the passage of relatively undiluted contrast medium directly to the cervical region. Exposures are then performed, as described under lateral C1–C2 puncture.

Thoracic myelography

As for cervical myelography, contrast medium may be introduced by lumbar or cervical routes. If a spinal block is suspected, a lumbar puncture can be performed and contrast medium introduced with the cranial end of the table tilted 10° head down. However, because of the normal thoracic kyphosis, contrast medium can not be made to pool in the thoracic region in the prone position. When the contrast medium has been manipulated to the cervico-dorsal region, the patient can be rapidly turned supine.

If a block is not suspected and maximum detail is required the more desirable technique is to perform a lateral C1–C2 puncture with the patient lying supine. The foot end of the table is then gently tipped down while the contrast medium is introduced, resulting in less dilution of the contrast medium (Gabrielsen et al 1980).

Total myelography

The clinical picture will dictate which technique is used. If a cervical lesion is considered clinically to be most likely lesion, then a lateral C1–C2 puncture in the prone position should be performed and the contrast medium directed caudally. If a lumbar or low thoracic lesion is thought more likely, the lumbar route with the patient prone may be used. In either case, the cervical and lumbar regions are examined in the prone position first and the patient is then turned supine for the thoracic segment of the examination.

Myelography with oily contrast media

Dosages:
1. 3 ml for diagnosis of spinal block
2. 12 ml for lumbar examination
3. 12–18 ml for thoracic and cervical examination

Technique

Because oily contrast media are not water miscible, the lumbar route may be used for all types of examination. An absolutely midline puncture, best obtained by prone puncture, is desirable to facilitate withdrawal of contrast medium at the end of the examination. If a spinal block is discovered and its upper limit needs delineation, the contrast medium can be introduced either by cisternal or lateral C1–C2 puncture. The contrast medium should be withdrawn completely at the end of the examination. This will necessitate a repuncture, following supine studies.

For visualization of the posterior aspect of the cord and the foramen magnum, the needle should be withdrawn and the patient turned supine. Any side-indicating markers on the serial changers should be resited appropriately. A cheap, useful method of indicating the degree and the direction of angulation of the patient at the time any radiograph is exposed is the taping of an ampoule of oily contrast medium directly onto the serial changer, alongside the mandatory side marker.

Posterior fossa myelography

In the era of nuclear magnetic resonance imaging and CT with low dose water soluble contrast media, posterior fossa myelography with either oily or water soluble contrast medium cannot be justified, because of the likelihood of adverse reactions and complications.

Complications of myelography

The complications can be divided into those due to needle puncture and those due to the contrast medium itself.

Complications of needle puncture

Lumbar puncture
1. Posture dependent headache, nausea and vomiting are probably due to continued CSF leakage.
2. Direct damage to the conus medullaris may result from puncture performed cranial to the L3–L4 disc level.

Lateral C1–C2 puncture. Direct puncture of the cord, with or without injection of contrast medium into the cord substance, can result in neurological deficit and even death.

Cisternal puncture. Direct puncture of the medulla can result in permanent neurological deficit or death.

Adverse reactions to contrast media

Oily contrast media. By far the most feared side effect is arachnoiditis. This varies from asymptomatic obliteration of nerve root sheaths to extensive adhesions, involving cauda equina and the spinal cord itself, which can result in a crippling, painful and progressive paraparesis and death. Arachnoiditis in the basal cisterns induced by oily contrast media has resulted in the development of obstructive, non-communicating hydrocephalus and death. This potential complication has been the main stimulus for the development of water soluble contrast media.

Water soluble contrast media. Most of the data concerning adverse reactions to water soluble contrast media relates to metrizamide. Although it has not been shown to induce arachnoiditis in clinically used concentrations and volumes, it has a number of other side effects. The most serious of these include:
1. Convulsions.
2. Aseptic meninigitis, which in turn may be associated with confusion, disorientation and psychosensory disorders, all of which are temporary.
3. Motor deficits reported include monoplegia, hemiplegia and aphasia.
4. Sensory deficits include visual and auditory loss.
5. Myoclonus, meningismus, hyperreflexia and areflexia are usually due to central nervous system irritation and are transient. Much more common (approximately 50% of patients) are headache, nausea and vomiting.

Prevention of complications

The use of water soluble contrast media whenever possible will eliminate the development of arachnoiditis. If oily contrast media have to be used, they should be removed completely at the end of the examination by siphoning or gentle suction, preferably through the cannula insert of a Cuatico needle. The use of intrathecal corticosteroids, which may themselves produce an arachnoiditic reaction, is positively contraindicated.

As water soluble contrast media reactions are in part dose related, the minimal possible concentration and total volume should be used.

Hydration of the patient is vital. Oral fluids should be continued to within 2 hours of the procedure and recommenced immediately after. Even routine intravenous fluids have been recommended (Potts et al 1977), but these should be used only if adequate oral hydration cannot be achieved.

Withdrawal of water soluble contrast medium at the completion of the examination has also been recommended (Hurwitz et al 1980), but no more than half of the contrast medium can be recovered, due to its miscibility with CSF. Furthermore, a considerable quantity of CSF has also to be withdrawn in order to retrieve contrast media, so the benefits of this method are outweighed by its disadvantages. As a general rule, the less interference there is with the patient and subarachnoid space, the better.

Although there is debate as to whether lying still, sitting, or actually walking around is the most appropriate post-procedural management, there is general agreement that the head should be raised at least 30° relative to the lower back to minimize the concentration of contrast medium in contact with the cerebrum. This usually requires postoperative orders stipulating 6 hours of head elevation. It is wise, also, to instruct the patient as to why this position is important for his well being, and to emphasize the need for a high fluid intake.

For any study involving the thoracic and cervical regions the importance of horizontal beam screening cannot be over emphasized, particularly as an aid to a cervical myelogram performed via a lateral C1–C2 puncture. It is only with horizontal beam screening that the head of the contrast medium column can be localized and controlled.

Relative contraindications to the use of water soluble contrast media in the subarachnoid space include a known history of epilepsy and current phenothiazine and tricyclic antidepressant drug therapy.

DISCOGRAPHY

Indications

1. The evaluation of severe low back pain and sciatica after normal lumbar CT and myelography.
2. When fusion of vertebrae is to be performed discography of the adjacent disc spaces should be performed to ensure that they are sufficiently healthy to cope with the inevitable additional stress.
3. As an adjunct to chemonucleolysis of intervertebral discs.

Materials

Four sets of discogram needles, consisting of 18 gauge guides with inner 22 gauge puncture needles, should be readily available. Water soluble non-ionic contrast media (Iopamidol, Iohexol) in concentrations of iodine of the order of 240–300 mg/ml are used. A metal enclosed glass 10 ml luerlock syringe, to enable the safe application of pressure, and local anaesthetic complete the basic requirements.

Technique

Lumbar discography

Both oblique and direct posterior approaches may be used. The oblique approach avoids puncture of the lumbar theca.

Oblique approach.* The level of the required disc space is established by screening. Local anaesthetic is injected into the epidermis and dermis one average hand's breadth from the midline, near to the lateral border of the sacrospinalis group of muscles. Under screening control and with the patient lying prone the guide needle is directed obliquely anteriorly and medially to a point as near as possible to the posterolateral border of the disc (Fig. 5.21).

The inner 22 gauge needle is inserted through the 18 gauge guide into the disc nucleus. Entry is signalled by a sudden loss of resistance as force is applied to the needle. The adequacy of positioning of the needle point should be confirmed by AP and lateral radiographs. The tip should be more than 1 cm into the disc as injections into the annulus may produce both artefactual appearances and artefactual patient responses (Quinnell 1980).

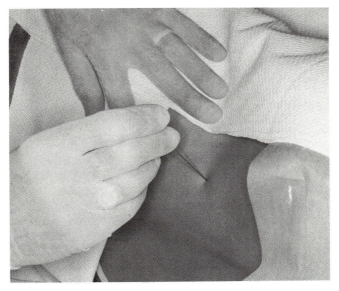

Fig. 5.21 Oblique approach for discography. Needle introduced at lateral border of sacrospinalis muscle group. Needle bevel down to induce upward curve of needle path.

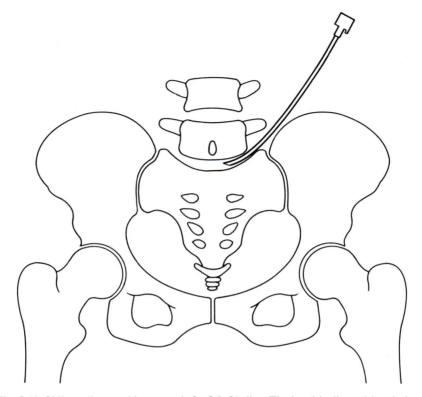

Fig. 5.22 Oblique discographic approach for L5–S1 disc. The bevel is directed interiorly to facilitate a curved needle path made necessary by the obstruction provided by the iliac wing.

Entry into the L5–S1 disc may require an inferiorly oblique approach and use of the needle bevel to 'bend' the needle in its course (Fig. 5.22). Alternatively the direct posterior approach may be necessary.

Direct posterior approach. With the patient in the left lateral position the guide needle is introduced in the midline to a point just deep to the ligamentum flavum. The fine central needle is passed slowly through the guide needle into the disc substance. The position of the needle tip within the nucleus pulposus is verified by AP and lateral radiographs.

Contrast medium injection

After advising the patient of the need to report accurately the nature and severity of any pain experienced, 0.5–2.0 ml of contrast medium is forcibly injected into the disc. Normal, healthy discs will absorb only approximately 0.5 ml, and considerable force is required. Degenerate discs will provide little resistance and receive a larger contrast medium volume. A maximum of 1.5–2.0 ml of contrast medium is injected.

CERVICAL DISCOGRAPHY

Indications

Cervical root pain, normal myelography.

Materials

As for lumbar discography, with the exception that the needle combination is a 22 gauge guide needle and a 26 gauge inner needle.

Technique

With the patient lying supine and head hyperextended, the carotid sheath is palpated and displaced laterally with the fingers and the trachea is displaced medially. Local anaesthetic is infiltrated into the overlying skin and the anterior longitudinal ligament at the level selected by fluoroscopy. The guide needle is passed obliquely to the anterior longitudinal ligament overlying the disc and the inner 26 gauge needle is inserted through the guide needle into the centre of the disc. After verification of the needle position by AP and lateral radiographs, contrast medium is injected and the patient's reactions recorded. A healthy disc will accept only up to 0.5 ml with an associated high resistance to injection.

The validity of cervical discography has been questioned even more than has that of lumbar discography. With the advent of CT and CT cisternography, there appears to be little indication for cervical discography.

PNEUMOENCEPHALOGRAPHY

With the development of CT, nuclear magnetic resonance imaging and non-ionic water soluble contrast media, pneumoencephalography, an elegant, but uncomfortable procedure with a significant morbidity, has been superseded and should no longer be performed. It will not be described in this book.

CT AIR CISTERNOGRAPHY

Indication

The diagnosis of intracanalicular acoustic and facial neurinomas.

Equipment

22 gauge, short-bevelled lumbar puncture needle. CT scanner, capable of performing thin (1–2 mm) scan slices.

Technique

Lumbar puncture is performed with the patient sitting on the CT scanner table with trunk flexed. Two or three pillows in the patient's lap and a sympathetic attendant to reassure and give support are helpful in maintaining the patient's compliance. The sitting position is the best position in which to puncture any patient in whom lumbar puncture has proven difficult in the prone or lateral position, no matter how severe the degree of spinal stenosis or kyphoscoliosis (G H du Boulay 1975). The interspinous space between L3 and L4 (the first space above the level of the iliac crests) is usually easily palpated. Because of the tautness of the stretched theca in the flexed sitting position, entry of the 22 gauge needle into the subarachnoid space is almost always signalled by a distinct 'give'. If the needle has been advanced no more than 2 mm at a time after piercing the ligamentum flavum, it should be advanced another 1 mm to ensure that the whole of the bevel is within the subarachnoid space. Te stylette is replaced and the patient is positioned in a reclining position with weight supported on the elbow opposite to the internal auditory canal which is to be examined. The axis of head and neck is parallel to that of the body with the face slightly rotated towards the table (Fig. 5.23).

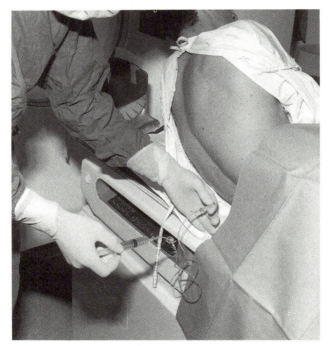

Fig. 5.23 CT air cisternography. The patient reclines on elbow with affected side up, while 3–5 ml of air is slowly injected through lumbar puncture needle.

After removal of a CSF specimen for laboratory examination, 3–5 ml of air is slowly injected through the needle. The patient is forewarned that he may experience a 'popping' sensation in the affected ear and a moderate headache. With the radiologist keeping the patient's head in the same position relative to the body, the patient reclines completely on the side opposite to that being examined. Scans of 1.5–2 mm are performed contiguously through the whole of the internal auditory canals and the resultant scans are processed using a bone algorithm and an expanded window width of 4000 Hounsfield units. If no air enters the canal, despite the pressure of air in the immediately contiguous cerebello-pontine angle cistern, the radiologist should firmly shake and slightly jar the patient's head to overcome any surface tension induced artefacts and repeat the scan. A normal study results when air fills the whole length of the internal auditory canal, outlining its neural and vascular contents.

Should it be desired to investigate the other internal auditory canal, this can usually be achieved by quickly rotating the patient's head through 180° in either direction and rescanning as above.

Complications

In approximately 50% of patients a moderately severe headache will follow immediately upon the introduction of the air. This is the only complication specific to the introduction of air. The standard post lumbar puncture complications may also occur.

Rest in bed for 24 hours is usually all that is required.

WATER SOLUBLE CONTRAST MEDIUM CISTERNOGRAPHY

The complications of introducing iodine into the cerebral subarachnoid space in concentrations sufficiently high to be visualized by conventional radiography or tomography are unacceptably high. Because of the ready availability of CT scanners, which can readily detect low subarachnoid concentrations of iodine, water soluble contrast medium cisternography should no longer be performed.

CT CISTERNOGRAPHY WITH WATER SOLUBLE CONTRAST MEDIA

Indications

1. Detection of low brain stem tumours.
2. Differentiation and delineation of intra-axial and extra-axial lesions in the posterior fossa.
3. Further evaluation of suprasellar masses.
4. Confirmation of the diagnosis of empty sella in equivocal cases.

5. Differentiation of subarachnoid space from subdural collections, arachnoid and parasitic cysts.
6. Determination of site of CSF leak.
7. Diagnosis of communicating hydrocephelus.

Materials

1. 22 gauge, short-bevelled lumbar puncture needle.
2. Non-ionic contrast media in concentrations of 200–240 mg iodine/ml.
3. Tilt table or tiltable trolley.

Technique

The same relative contraindications for water soluble contrast media in myelography apply.

A lumbar puncture with a 22 gauge disposable, short-bevelled needle is performed. This can be performed under screening control, as for myelography, but this is not necessary. A trolley capable of tilting up to 30° at one end may be used. Following lumbar puncture and removal of a small volume of CSF for laboratory analysis, 6 ml of non-ionic water soluble contrast medium is introduced into the lumbar theca and the needle is removed. If on a tilt table the patient may then be tilted 45° head down for 2 minutes, or the maximum angulation on a tilting trolley should be achieved. If the tilt trolley can be tilted only through an angle between 15° and 30°, the patient should be positioned on one side for 30 s and then the other, all the time maintaining the cranial tilt. This will overcome the problem of patients with gross kyphoscoliosis. After being brought back to the horizontal, the patient is ready for scanning.

Scans of 3–5 mm thickness are performed in the transverse axial position from the level of arch of C2 to 1 cm above the dorsum sellae. Sagittal reformations are useful. Images should be photographed at narrow and wide window widths, such as 350 and 1000 Hounsfield Units.

Complications

Because of the small quantity of contrast medium used, the complications are basically those of lumbar puncture. These can be minimized by the use of a lumbar puncture needle of calibre no greater than 22 gauge.

REFERENCES

Chakera T M H, Hartley D E 1982 Catheterization of tortuous carotid arteries. American Journal of Neuroradiology 3: 447.
Doyle T, Tress B 1983 Autotomography with metrizamide myelography: an aid to visualisation of the cranio-cervical junction and cerebellar tonsils. Clinical Radiology 34: 401–403

du Bonlay G H 1975 Personal communication

Earnest F. IV, Forbes G, Sandok B A et al 1983 Complications of cerebral angiography: prospective assessment of risk. American Journal of Neuroradiology 4: 1191–1197

Faught E, Trader S D, Hanna G R 1979 Cerebral complications of angiography for transient ischaemia and stroke: prediction of risk. Neurology (NY) 29: 4–15

Gabrielsen T O, Seeger J F, Knake J E, Burke D P, Stilwill E W 1980 C1 C2 puncture with the patient supine for thoracic metrizamide myelography. Radiology 136: 229–230

Grainger R G 1982 Intravascular radiological contrast media: the past, the present and the future. British Journal of Radiology 55: 1–18

Guinto F C Jr 1982 New catheter for tortuous vertebral artery. American Journal of Neuroradiology 3: 85–86

Hurwitz S R, Suydam G, Steinberg A 1980 Aspiration of metrizamide following lumbar myelography. Radiology 136: 789

Kerber C, Mani R L, Bank W O, Cromwell L D 1975 Selective cerebral angiography through the axillary artery. Neuroradiology 10: 131–135

Kerber C W, Cromwell L D, Drayer B P, Bank W O 1978 Cerebral ischaemia: I Current angiographic techniques, complications and safety. American Journal of Roentgenology 130: 1097–1103

Mani R L 1970 A new double-curve catheter for selective femoro-cerebral angiography. Radiology 94: 607–611

Mani R L, Eisenberg R L, McDonald E J Jr, Pollock J A, Mani Jr 1978 Complications of catheter cerebral arteriography: analysis of 5,000 procedures. I Criteria and incidence. American Journal of Roentgenology 131: 861–865

Olivecrona H 1977 Complications of cerebral angiography. Neuroradiology 14: 175–181

Orrison W W, Elderik O P, Sackett J F 1983 Lateral C1 C2 puncture for cervical myelography. Part III: Historical, anatomic, and technical considerations. Radiology 146: 401–408

Potts D G, Gomex D G, Abbott G A 1977 Possible causes of complications of myelography with water-soluble contrast media. Acta Radiologica (Suppl) 355: 390–401

Quinnell R C 1980 An investigation of artefacts in lumbar discography. British Journal of Radiology 53: 831–839

Sage M R 1983 Kinetics of water-soluble contrast media in the central nervous system. American Journal of Roentgenology 4: 897–906

Simmons C R, Tsao A C, Thompson J R 1973 Angiographic approach to the difficult aortic arch: a new technique for transfemoral cerebral angiography in the aged. American Journal of Roentgenology 119: 605–612

Willson J K V 1980 A new technique for cerebral angiography: the variable stiffness guidewire. Radiology 134: 427–430

6

Arthrography

TEMPOROMANDIBULAR JOINT (TMJ)

Indications

Temporomandibular pain and dysfunction, such as clicking and locking, are problems being increasingly recognized and treated by the dental profession. Arthrography is indicated to assess internal derangements of the joint, particularly anterior meniscal displacement with or without recapture on opening, perforation of the meniscus and osteoarthritis. The technique also offers the therapeutic option of steroid injection which may be of value in patients with rheumatoid arthritis.

Technique

The patient is placed on the side on a fluoroscopic table. The lower shoulder is elevated on a pad, the side being examined is uppermost; the head lies against the table top. The result, with a vertical beam, is to project the upper TMJ above the lower. The optimal degree of head rotation is selected fluoroscopically. The skin anterior to the ear is cleansed and infiltrated with 1% lignocaine down to the condyle. A suitable contrast medium is meglumine sodium diatrizoate 60%. To 10 ml of contrast, 0.5 ml of 1:1000 adrenaline is added. In order to avoid overdistension of the joint no more than 0.5 ml should be injected. With the mouth a little open, a 2.5 cm long 25 gauge needle is passed down to touch the postero-superior part of the head of the mandible. The needle tip is moved gradually posteriorly until it is felt to slip behind the condyle. If the needle is in the lower joint space it will move forward and back with the condyle as the mouth is opened and closed. Under fluoroscopy, a small amount of contrast is injected and should pass rapidly over the top of the condyle to appear anterior to it (Figs 6.1 and 6.2).

An adequate amount of contrast is usually 0.2–0.3 ml and more than this has a tendency to leak out of the joint when the needle is withdrawn, thereby obscuring the structures. When the needle is withdrawn, the optimal position of the head is selected and spot films are taken with the

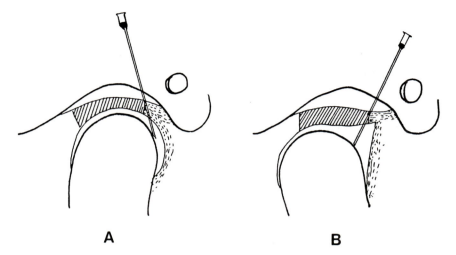

Fig. 6.1 (A) Shows the optimal insertion point for the needle in the lower TMJ space. (B) When the mouth is opened a little a correctly positioned needle moves forward with the mandibular condyle.

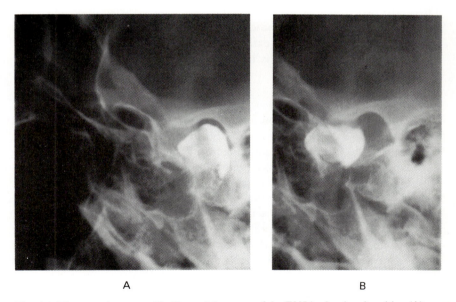

Fig. 6.2 The normal contrast filled lower joint space of the TMJ in the closed position (A) covers the condylar head like a shower cap. When the mouth is opened (B) the posterior part of the space takes on a tented appearance.

mouth open and closed, before and after any click. Contrast appearing in the upper joint space indicates a meniscal perforation and early fluoroscopy may be required to see this.

Difficulties

1. If the lower joint space cannot be entered it is important to have the mouth open a little. As the mandibular condyle moves forward, the lower joint space opens up posteriorly, thus allowing a larger volume for needle puncture.
2. Contrast extravasation can be avoided by carefully screening the initial injection. If contrast does not flow rapidly over the condylar head, the needle tip must be repositioned. Overdistension of the joint must also be avoided.
3. If the condylar head cannot be touched with the 2.5 cm long 25G needle, the 3.5 cm long 23G needle should be used. This problem occasionally arises in large patients with plump cheeks.

SPINAL APOPHYSEAL JOINTS

Indications

There are two principal uses for apophyseal joint arthrography, one diagnostic and the other therapeutic. Degenerative change can be shown by demonstrating deformity and extravasation from the synovial joint capsule. Therapeutic steroid injection is helpful in some patients.

Technique

The patient is placed prone on a fluoroscopic table with the trunk rotated 45° toward the side to be injected. The lower three apophyseal joints on the rotated side can now be identified en face and their surface marking fixed by a local anaesthetic needle infiltrating the skin superficially. At each joint a 22 gauge spinal needle is passed vertically down under fluoroscopic control into the posterior aspect of the joint. To diagnose degenerative change, 0.5 ml of contrast, 60% urographic (meglumine sodium diatrizoate) is injected. The reproduction of pain symptoms on injection of particular joints confirms that they are the cause of pain. Contrast medium is used since extravasation outside the joint capsule is said to represent significant degenerative change in the joint. This is disputed, however, since it is probably quite easy to overdistend the joint and rupture it.

Therapeutic injection of the apophyseal joints, for a patient with known symptomatic degeneration, is worth a trial. A mixture of equal parts of steroid such as Depomedrol and local anaesthetic such as 2% xylocaine can be injected, 0.5 ml inside and 0.5 ml outside each joint capsule.

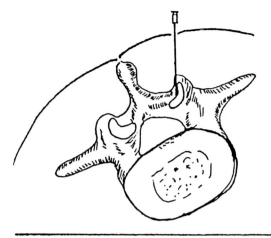

Fig. 6.3 With the patient's trunk rotated 45° elevating the side to be injected, the apophyseal joint can be entered by a vertical approach under fluoroscopy.

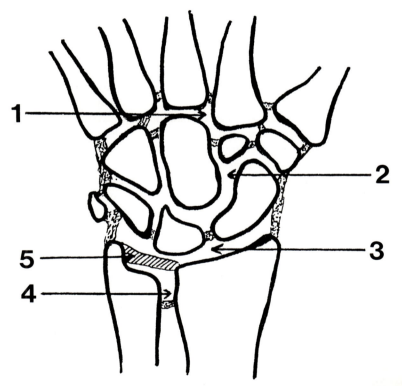

Fig. 6.4 The compartments of the wrist joint: (1) The carpometacarpal. (2) The mid carpal. (3) The radiocarpal. (4) The inferior radio-ulnar spaces. (5) The ulnocarpal fibro cartilage. The point of needle insertion for arthrography is at (3).

WRIST JOINT

This procedure is only rarely performed. In rheumatoid arthritis it may demonstrate synovial proliferation as nodular irregularity of the contrast outline. In trauma, contrast may extravasate from the radiocarpal joint, communicate with other compartments or outline tendon sheaths.

Technique

The hand is placed prone on a fluoroscopic table and the dorsum of the wrist is sterilized, draped and infiltrated with local anaesthetic. Under fluoroscopic control a 23 gauge needle is introduced into the radiocarpal joint from the dorsal side. This is usually made easier by having the wrist flexed over a small pad. 2 ml of 60% meglumine sodium diatrizoate is injected and if the needle is correctly placed this should flow rapidly away from the tip. AP lateral and oblique films are obtained. The normal radiocarpal joint is separated from the inferior radio-ulnar cavity by a triangular fibrocartilage. Communication with the inferior radio-ulnar and with the mid-carpal joints occur as occasional normal variants.

HIP JOINT

In adults the main indication for this technique is the demonstration of loosening of hip prostheses, in which case contrast may be seen extending between the femoral component and the bone. It may, however, be used to evaluate the articular cartilage in patients with rheumatoid or osteoarthritis. Iliopsoas bursae and synovial cysts may be demonstrated since these may present as inguinal swellings. In children it is of much greater value. In Perthes disease the true shape of the femoral head can be determined, and its relationship to the acetabular fossa. In congenital dislocation of the hip it is important to demonstrate the presence of a fibro-cartilaginous limbus between the femoral head and the acetabulum, since this may interfere with reduction of the hip.

Technique

Initial plain films, AP and lateral are obtained. With the patient supine, a point at the junction of the femoral head and neck is selected fluoroscopically and infiltrated with 1% lignocaine. The surface marking of this point is 3 cm at right angles inferior to the mid-point of the inguinal ligament.

After routine skin preparation, a 22G spinal needle is passed vertically down to puncture the joint capsule at this point. If a 'give' is not felt on passing through the capsule, the needle should be advanced down until the periosteum of bone is felt. A small amount of contrast, e.g. 60% meglumine sodium diatrizoate, is injected and if the needle is correctly placed this

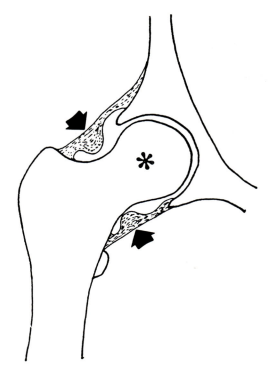

Fig. 6.5 Outline of the hip joint showing the impression of the zona orbicularis (arrows) into the joint space. The star is at the point of injection for an arthrogram.

will flow away from the tip. In all 5 ml of contrast will be injected. AP and lateral films are obtained, with obliques if necessary. The normal hip joint space extends down the femoral neck almost to the intertrochanteric line. The joint space is compressed by the zona orbicularis, formed by the deep fibres of the ischiofemoral ligament. These fibres encircle the femoral neck and give a circumferential filling defect in the contrast.

If the procedure is for evaluation of a hip prosthesis a modification of the standard technique is employed to use subtraction. This is to subtract out the metal prosthesis and the surrounding glue, in order to see small amounts of contrast leakage around the loosened femoral or acetabular prosthesis. The position of the needle is as for a normal hip arthrogram. The spinal needle is passed down to the head of the hip prosthesis until metal contact is made. The leg is then immobilized and on AP film is made for use as a subtraction mask. Now 15–20 ml of contrast are injected into the joint space. Postoperatively this space is considerably larger than normal. With the leg still immobilized a second AP film is taken for the subtraction study.

In an infant or child preoperative sedation is necessary. The needle entry point is 1 cm inferior to the neck epiphyseal plate between the femoral head and neck and 1 cm medial to the lateral margin of the femoral neck. A 22 gauge spinal needle is suitable and 1–2 ml of contrast are instilled.

KNEE JOINT

Indications

The principal uses of knee arthrography are the diagnosis of meniscus damage and the presence of a ruptured Baker's cyst in the differential diagnosis of acute calf pain. Arthrography may also be useful in assessing injury, especially of the cruciate ligaments and osteochondritis dissecans.

Contraindications

Arthrography should not be performed on any joint in the presence of an overlying skin infection. Bleeding tendency or anti-coagulant therapy are relative contraindications. Allergic reactions at arthrography are very rare, most probably because of the slow absorption of the small doses involved. However, the procedure should not be performed on patients with previous history of significant allergic reaction.

Technique

Plain films should be obtained routinely especially in post trauma cases, in order to identify loose bodies in the joint. Frontal, lateral and intercondylar views are routine. Plain films may indicate the presence of an effusion. If the width of the supra patella bursa in the lateral view is greater than 10 mm, fluid is usually present, and if less than 5 mm, usually absent (Gilula 1977). The plain films will also serve to determine the best radiographic exposure factors. The knee is sterilized and draped. A point on the mid-lateral margin of the patella is infiltrated with local anaesthetic and an 18 gauge needle is inserted posterior to the patella at this point.

Entry can be made easier if the knee is extended and relaxed and the patella pulled laterally by the operator. All joint fluid is aspirated both for diagnostic examination and because any remaining fluid will dilute the contrast medium. A mixture of 3 ml of 60% meglumine sodium diatrizoate, 1 ml of 2% lignocaine and 0.5 ml 1:1000 adrenaline is injected. Correct needle placement is determined by the fact that the first ml of contrast mixture will flow away from the needle tip, usually to the medial knee joint space. Room air is injected into the joint until discomfort is felt, up to a maximum of about 50 ml. The patient is now placed prone on the fluoroscopic table after mild exercise of the knee. Tangential films are taken of the anterior, mid and posterior parts of each meniscus with appropriate distracting stress to open up the joint space. Stress is applied in a valgus direction for the medial meniscus and in a varus direction for the lateral.

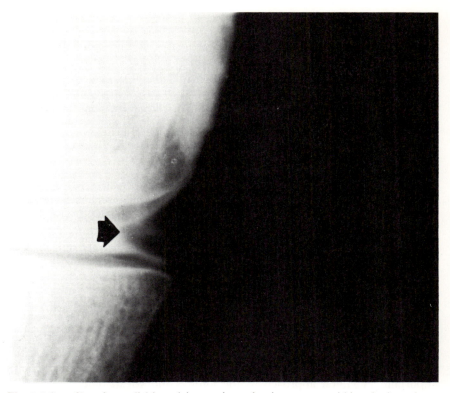

Fig. 6.6 Spot film of a medial knee joint meniscus showing contrast within a horizontal tear (arrow).

A variety of mechanical devices have been described to facilitate this (Lee & Sanders 1978). A total of 6 to 12 spot films should be taken of each meniscus. Films may be taken with a fluoroscopic film changer provided a focal spot of less than 1 mm is available. The previously determined exposure factors may be used since a phototimer will usually give unsatisfactorily over exposed films. While coning is important it should be wide enough to include the whole joint space being examined, i.e. the medial half of the joint for the medial meniscus. This also allows better orientation when interpreting the films. Great care should also be taken in labelling the films as to side and position.

A lateral film with stress to demonstrate the anterior cruciate ligament is now taken. This is obtained by holding ankle steady and pushing the upper tibia forward, while the patient lies laterally on the table with the knee flexed 90°. This manoeuvre will stress the anterior cruciate ligament which runs from the anterior tibial spine to the medial aspect of the lateral femoral condyle. The anterior cruciate ligament may be better demonstrated by lateral tomography.

The joint cavity may be divided by several incomplete synovial folds called plicae. These are best demonstrated by a final routine AP and lateral film of the extended knee. The posterior aspect of the joint is normally smooth but in rheumatoid arthritis may exhibit a Baker's cyst with posterior leakage. This can be demonstrated by injecting 10 ml of contrast and local anaesthetic mixture together with 10–20 ml of air. Stress views are not taken but adequate lateral views of the calf should be obtained to show the inferior extent of the leak.

ELBOW JOINT

The elbow arthrogram may be single or double contrast. Single contrast studies are useful in identifying capsular ruptures. Enlargement of the joint space may be seen in joint effusion, rheumatoid arthritis, where the synovium has a saccular appearance and pigmented villonodular synovitis, where a filling defect will be seen. Double contrast studies are indicated to identify osteochonditis dissecans, chondromatosis and the intra- or extra-capsular position of bone fragments.

Technique

Initial plain films, in the lateral projection, to identify displacement of the fat pads anterior and posterior to the distal humerus indicating joint effusion, and in the AP projection to identify loose bone fragments are most important. A lateral approach to the joint is the safest. The head of the

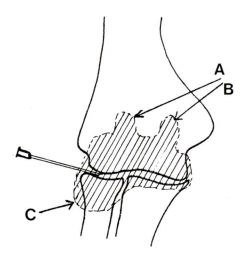

Fig. 6.7 Anterior view of the elbow showing the correct needle position. (A) and (B) represent the normal superior recesses of the joint space and (C) the recess around the head of the radius.

radius can be palpated by pronation and supination of the hand. The groove just proximal to this is infiltrated with 1% lignocaine. A 21 gauge needle is inserted here into the joint space between the head of the radius and the capitellum. Any joint fluid present is aspirated and 5 ml of meglumine sodium diatrizoate 60% is injected under fluoroscopic control. If the needle is in the joint space the contrast will flow rapidly away from the tip. For a double contrast study 1 ml of contrast and 10 ml of room air are injected. Films are obtained in the AP, lateral and both oblique projections.

Pitfalls

The normal processes of the elbow joint space are upwards anterior and posterior to the distal humerus and also downwards around the neck of the radius in the membrana sacciformis deep to the supinator muscle. In rheumatoid arthritis contrast medium may appear in the peri-articular lymphatics (Weston 1969b).

SHOULDER JOINT

Indications

The most commonly diagnosed conditions at shoulder arthrography are partial or complete tears of the rotator cuff, capsular tears from recurrent dislocations and the small capsule of adhesive capsulitis. Arthrography is

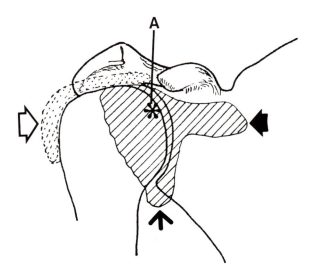

Fig. 6.8 Anterior view of the shoulder arthrogram. The normal subscapularis (broad arrow) and inferior recesses (fine arrow) are shown. The position of abnormal contrast extravasation into the subacromion and subdeltoid bursae (open arrow), indicates a rotator cuff tear. The star at (A) indicates the injection point.

a useful procedure in all patients with chronic shoulder pain where the cause is not clear. In some cases an arthrogram may be therapeutic in breaking down the adhesions of capsulitis.

Technique

Preliminary films of the shoulder are taken in the AP projection with the humerus in internal and external rotation, and in the infero-superior projection. These are taken to identify calcifications in the supraspinatus tendon and other soft tissues. With the patient supine and the arm in external rotation, the anterior aspect of the shoulder is sterilized and draped. The skin and subcutaneous tissue is infiltrated with 1% lignocaine at a point 2 cm below and lateral to the coracoid process. This should mark the mid-point of the glenohumeral joint and is checked fluoroscopically with the local needle in situ. A 21 gauge needle is now advanced vertically down into the joint at this spot, injecting lignocaine until a change in resistance is felt. If the needle is in the correct place in the joint, a test injection of 0.5 ml of contrast will be seen to flow away from the needle tip. Suitable contrast medium is 60% meglumine sodium diatrizoate mixed with an equal volume of lignocaine. This reduces the hypertonicity of the contrast and reduces post procedural pain. For a single contrast study 15 ml of the above mixture are injected. For a double contrast study 5 ml of contrast mixture are injected together with 0.5 ml of 1:1000 adrenaline to delay resorption. This is followed by 10 ml of room air. The shoulder is exercised for a few minutes and the routine films are taken. These are AP views in internal and external rotation, both with 15° of caudal beam angulation to project the supraspinatus tendon away from the acromion process. An axillary view and possibly one of the bicipital groove may be obtained. In a double contrast study, erect films both in internal and external rotation with a sandbag in the hand to pull the humeral head down from the acromion and glenoid, are obtained.

The single contrast technique is best for adhesive capsulitis studies and the double contrast for rotation cuff tears and cartilage abnormalities. The axillary view is best to demonstrate the glenoid labrum, which is shown as a triangular soft tissue density.

Pitfalls

It is normal to see contrast extending into the synovial sheath of biceps long head in the bicipital groove. The subscapularis bursa normally communicates with the shoulder joint also. This bursa, lying deep to subscapularis muscle, is best seen in the axillary view. While it is well seen in internal rotation it tends to be obliterated on external rotation because of the tenseness of the subscapularis muscle. The appearance of contrast in the subcromion bursa, however, indicates a rotator cuff tear.

ARTHROGRAPHY OF THE ANKLE

Indications

Most arthrograms of the ankle are performed to detect tears of lateral collateral ligament. A few are done to detect intra-articular loose bodies and to assess the articular cartilage.

Technique

Initial plain films are taken to assess the position of any bone fragments. The anterior aspect of the joint is sterilized and draped. The path of the dorsalis pedis artery is determined and the area medial to this is infiltrated with 1% xylocaine. A 3 cm long 21 gauge needle is introduced into the medial third of the tibio-talar joint under fluoroscopic control. It is best to angle the needle slightly cranially to avoid the overhanging anterior margin of the tibia.

Any fluid inside the joint is aspirated and 6–10 ml of 60% meglumine sodium diatrizoate together with a small amount of 1% xylocaine are injected. The needle is correctly placed if the contrast flows rapidly away from the tip. Injection is continued until pressure is felt or the full 10 ml of contrast mixture is injected. The ankle is exercised as vigorously as practicable and AP, lateral and external oblique films are obtained.

The examination should be performed within 72 hours of injury if the aim is to detect ligamentous tears. After this time delay, false negative results may be obtained.

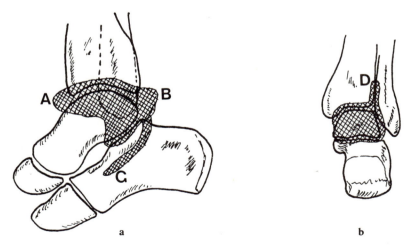

a

b

Fig. 6.9 (a) Lateral view of the normal ankle arthrogram, showing the anterior recess (A), the posterior recess (B), and flexor digitorum tendon sheath (C).
(b) Frontal view of the ankle showing the normal inferior tibio fibular recess (D) of the joint space.

Normal appearance

There are three normal outpouchings of the ankle joint. In the lateral view there are anterior and posterior smooth walled recesses, and on the AP view an interosseous recess between the distal tibia and fibula. In approximately 10% of cases the tibio-talar joint communicates with the subtalar joint posteriorly. In 20% of cases there may be a normal communication with the tendon sheaths of flexor digitorum longus or flexor hallucis longus. Visualization of the peroneal tendon sheaths on the lateral side of the ankle, or extravasation of contrast into the soft tissues, both indicate a tear in the calcaneo-fibular ligament.

BURSOGRAPHY AND SMALL JOINT ARTHROGRAPHY

These procedures are not commonly performed. The interested reader is referred to the published work of W. J. Weston (1969a & b, 1970a, b & c, 1973), the principal authority in this area, and also Weston & Antilla (1972) and Weston & Palmer (1979).

REFERENCES

Gilula J A 1977 A simplified stress device for knee arthrography. Radiology 122: 828–829
Lee H R, Sanders W F 1978 A practical stress device for knee arthrography. Radiology 127:542
Weston W J 1969a The normal arthrograms of the metacarpophalangeal, metatarsophalangeal and interphalangeal joints. Australasian Radiology 13: 211
Weston W J 1969b Positive contrast arthrography of the normal mid tarsal joints. Australasian Radiology 13: 365
Weston W J 1970a The olecranon bursa. Australasian Radiology 14: 323
Weston W J 1970b The bursa deep to gluteus medius and minimus. Australasian Radiology 14:325
Weston W J 1970c The bursa deep to the Achilles tendon. Australasian Radiology 14: 327
Weston W J 1973 The deep infrapatellar bursa. Australasian Radiology 17: 212
Weston W J, Antilla P 1972 Synovial lesions of the mid tarsal and posterior subtaloid joints in rheumatoid arthritis. Australasian Radiology 16: 84
Weston W J, Palmer D G 1979 Soft tissues of the extremities. Springer-Verlag, New York

FURTHER READING

Ala-Ketola L, Puranen J, Koivisto E, Puupera M 1977 Arthrography in the diagnosis of ligamentous injuries and classification of ankle injuries. Radiology 125: 63–68
Andrew L, Lundberg B J 1965 Treatment of rigid shoulders by joint distension during arthrography. Acta Orthopaedica Scandinavica 36: 45–53
Astley R 1967 Arthrography in congenital dislocation of the hip. Clinical Radiology 18:253
Dalinka M K, Turner M L, Osterman A L, Batra Poonam 1981 Wrist arthrography. Radiologic Clinics of North America 19 (No 2) 217–226.
De Smet A A, Ting Y M, Weis J J 1975 Shoulder arthrography in rheumatoid arthritis. Radiology 116: 601–605
Debnam J W, Staple T W 1974 Arthrography of the knee after meniscectomy. Radiology 113: 67–71

Doyle T 1983 Arthrography of the temporomandibular joint, a simple technique. Clinical Radiology 34: 147–151

Doyle T, Hase M 1983 The clicking painful temporomandibular joint. Medical Journal of Australia 1: 17–21

Eto R T, Anderson P W, Harley P N 1975 Elbow arthrography with application of tomography. Radiology 115: 283–288

Gelman M I, Dunn H K 1976 Radiology of knee joint replacement. American Journal of Roentgenology 127: 447–455

Ghelman B, Doherty J H 1978 Demonstration of spondylolysis by arthrography of the apophyseal joints. American Journal of Roentgenology 130: 986–987

Ghelman B, Goldman A B 1977 The double contrast shoulder arthrogram: evaluation of rotatory cuff tears. Radiology 124: 251–254

Goldman A B, Ghelman B 1978 The double contrast shoulder arthrogram. Radiology 127: 655–663

Goldman A B, Katz M C, Freiberger R H 1975 Post traumatic adhesive capsulitis of the ankle. Arthrographic diagnosis. American Journal of Roentgenology 125: 585–588

Hall F M 1976 Pitfalls in knee arthrography. Radiology 118: 55–62

Hall F M 1981 Methodology in knee arthrography. Radiologic Clinics of North America 19 (No 2) 269–275

Harrison M D, Freiberger R H, Ranawat C S 1971 Arthrography of the rheumatoid wrist joint. American Journal of Roentgenology 112: 380–486

Katzberg R N, Dolwick M F, Helms C A 1980 Arthrotomography of the temporomandibular joint. American Journal of Roentgenology 134: 995–1003

Lapayowker M S, Cliff M M, Tourtellotte C D 1970 Arthrography in the diagnosis of cuff pain. Radiology 95: 319–323

McIntyre J L 1972 Arthrography of the lateral meniscus. Radiology 105: 531–536

Mittler S, Freiberger M J, Harrison-Stubbs M 1972 A method of improved cruciate ligament visualisation in double contrast arthrography. Radiology 102: 331–442

Montgomery C E 1974 Synovial recesses in knee arthrography. American Journal of Roentgenology 121: 86–88

Olson R W 1981 Ankle arthrography. Radiologic Clinics of North America 19 (No 2) 255–268

Pavlov H, Ghelman B G, Warren R F 1979 Double contrast arthrography of the elbow. Radiology 130: 87–95

Prager R J, Mall J C 1976 Arthrographic diagnosis of synovial chondromatosis. American Journal of Roentgenology 127: 344–346

Resnick D 1974 Radiology of the talo-calcaneal articulations: anatomic considerations and arthrography. Radiology 111: 581–586

Resnick D 1975 The roentgenographic anatomy of the tendon sheaths of the hand and wrist: tenography. American Journal of Roentgenology 124: 44–51

Salman M I 1976 Arthrography in total hip prosthesis complications. American Journal of Roentgenology 126: 743–750

Schwarz A M, Goldberg M J 1978 Hip arthrography in children. Skeletal Radiology 3: 155

Staple T W 1972 Arthrographic demonstration of ilio psoas bursa extension of the hip joint. Radiology 102: 515–516

7

Other miscellaneous practical procedures

PERCUTANEOUS ABSCESS DRAINAGE

Indications

This technique offers an increasingly viable alternative to surgical drainage in selected cases. The site and extent of the abscess must first be established by conventional radiography, ultrasound, radionuclide gallium scanning or CT. When the presence of an abscess is likely, CT is the diagnostic modality of choice (Gerzof et al 1981; Martin et al 1982; Van Sonnenberg et al 1982).

Suitability of abscesses for percutaneous drainage

Cavity shape. The most suitable is a well defined, unilocular cavity. Non-liquified necrosis of organs such as liver, spleen and pancreas, are not suitable.

Aetiology. Abscesses caused by most organisms are suitable, but those caused by hydatid disease must be avoided because of the risk of fatal anaphylaxis if the cyst contents are split. Aseptic collections, such as urinoma, lymphocoele and pancreatic pseudocyst may be drained as a single stage procedure. If a catheter is left in such an aseptic cavity, it should be for no longer than 24 hours. After this time the risk of secondary infection increases.

Access

It is most important to plan the safest access route. Ideally this should be the shortest and most direct one possible. However, intervening organs or vital structures, especially bowel, must not lie in the access path.

Equipment

Two catheter systems are widely used:
1. An 8–10F multiple side hole pigtail biliary drainage catheter which may

be replaced after a few days with a larger 12F Argyll catheter for better drainage.

2. The Ring-McLean sump drainage tube (Cook Inc.). This is a wide bore 12F flexible tube. A separate inner lumen allows air passage to the distal tip of the catheter resulting in a free flow of fluid and a reduction of negative pressure in the abscess. This prevents the cavity collapsing into the drain holes when suction is applied to the main tube. There is a side arm opening to allow flushing of the air lumen (Fig. 7.1).

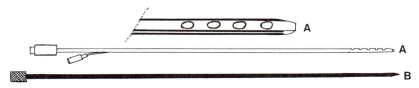

Fig. 7.1 The Ring-McLean sump drainage set including (A) the sump catheter, shown here with a magnified view of the tip section and (B) an inner stiffened trocar.

Technique

1. CT guidance is highly desirable since this will assure the operator that no vital structures are being traversed.
2. An ideal CT slice is selected which shows the optimal access route.
3. The patient is positioned at this slice level in the scanning gantry and the gantry laser light will mark the skin level. A small skin needle is placed on the proposed entry site and the patient is rescanned at this level.
4. When this slice including the skin marker appears on the display console, a cursor is placed on the skin marker, and another in the middle of the abscess. The computer is asked the distance between the two points (i.e. the depth of the abscess from the skin) and also the angle of the proposed access route from the vertical.
5. The skin is infiltrated with local anaesthetic and an exploratory, long 18G needle is passed down to the abscess along these coordinates and pus is aspirated for culture.
6. If a pigtail drain catheter is to be used, an 0.89 mm diameter (0.035 in) 80 cm broad J tipped guidewire is passed down to the cavity. The track is dilated to 10F and the drain tube is passed down to the abscess.
7. If the broader Ring-McLean sump drain is to be used, the tube is stiffened with an inner trocar. After the skin entry has been infiltrated well with local anaesthetic and a generous skin incision made, the sump drain is passed down over its trocar to the abscess along the predetermined coordinates.
8. The catheter should be fixed in position with a skin suture.

POST DRAINAGE MANAGEMENT

Irrigation

The catheter should be flushed every 6 hours with saline. If the pus is very thick, it can be liquified by instillation of a mucolytic agent Mucomyst (acetyl cysteine). Small volumes up to 5 ml of 10–20% solution are used, with each catheter flush.

Exchanges

The catheter position or the entire catheter may be changed if it is not performing adequately. Often this is because it is not lying in the most dependent part of the cavity to give maximum drainage.

Problems

1. The catheter becomes clogged. This is likely when there is resistance to irrigation. The cure for the problem is either repeated flushing of the tube with saline, or catheter replacement.
2. Poor response to catheter drainage. The usual causes are loculations, multiple abscesses or fistulae. Any of these problems may require a second catheter for optimum drainage.

FLUOROSCOPIC PERCUTANEOUS LUNG BIOPSIES

Indications

1. To gain diagnostic tissue for cytologic diagnosis from a lung mass.
2. To aspirate fluid for culture from a suspected lung abscess.
3. To gain lung tissue for microscopic examination in cases of mycotic lung infection such as aspergillosis.

Contraindications

1. The likelihood of a rounded lung mass being a hydatid cyst must be excluded. Puncture of such cysts may lead to anaphylaxis.
2. The likelihood of a mass being an arteriovenous malformation must be excluded by close inspection of the plain films.
3. Masses close to major vascular structures. should not have biopsies attempted.

Equipment

Of the many needles available the author's preference will be described. The 20G Surgimed Rotex is a screw type biopsy needle. Its advantage is

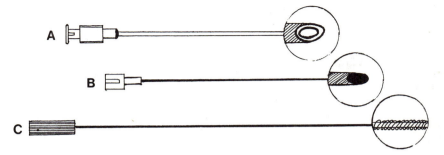

Fig. 7.2 The Surgimed Rotex (Cook Inc.) biopsy needle set, comprising a 20G sheath needle (A), with its trocar (B), the trocar is later replaced in the sheath needle by the inner screwthread needle (C).

that it provides cytological material which is less damaged than that from aspiration biopsies and also tissue fragments for histology. It comprises an inner needle with a screw tip, and an outer sheath with a cutting tip through which a trocar fits (Fig. 7.2).

Technique

1. The mass must be visible on both the AP and lateral views.
2. Biplane AP and lateral fluoroscopy is highly desirable otherwise the patient will need to be rolled on the fluoroscopy table.
3. The patient lies prone or supine on the table depending on the proximity of the mass to the front or back wall of the chest.
4. The skin vertically above the mass is sterilized, draped and infiltrated with local anaesthetic down to, but not through, the pleura.
5. The Rotex needle with its trocar in place is run vertically down to the anterior margin of the mass and the position checked in two views at right angles.
6. The inner trocar is removed and the screw needle is advanced to replace it. In suspended respiration this is screwed into the mass. As the screw needle is held firm, the outer cutting sheath is advanced over the screw, thereby slicing off the core of tissue held on the screw.
7. The whole assembly is removed and immediately the tissue from the screw is plated onto glass slides by a waiting technician, and fixed in 95% alcohol.

Complications

1. A chest film in expiration is performed routinely after the procedure to exclude a pneumothorax which will occur in about 5% of cases.
2. The incidence of pneumothorax can be considerably reduced by making only one needle pass through the pleura. Therefore, if the needle tip

requires repositioning, changes of direction should be made without withdrawing the needle so far that it comes out of the pleura.

CT GUIDED BIOPSIES

Indications

CT guided biopsy is now providing diagnostic information that was previously only available at the time of operation. The tissue yield is high and the risks are low.

Equipment

There are many styles of needle available.
1. The Chiba needle, 22 or 23G can be used for aspiration of tissue. It is very flexible and hard to control.
2. The Greene aspiration needle is available in 18–22G. It has the potential for obtaining a tissue core. It is most useful when little movement of the needle tip is possible as is required with the Rotex needle. Thus the Greene needle is more useful in the retroperitoneum and close to major structures.
3. The Rotex (Surgimed) is a 21G needle where a tissue piece held on the screw is sliced off by the outer cutting sheath. It has the potential to collect tissue fragments as well as cells for cytology. It appears to damage tissue specimens less than true aspiration needles but requires some movement of the tip. It is less useful near major blood vessels therefore.
4. The Tru-cut (Travenol) is a cutting biopsy needle. 14 or 16G. This produces a large core of tissue for histological study. Its large bore limits its usefulness to large solid organs.

Technique

1. The lesion to be biopsied is identified.
2. A scan showing the lesion is studied to find the optimum access route for the biopsy needle. This will avoid major structures including the bowel. The stomach may be traversed by a 21G needle en route to the pancreas, however.
3. Once the optimum access route is identified, a skin metal marker is placed over it and the patient scanned at that level.
4. When the image of the slice including the skin marker appears on the display console, a cursor is placed over the marker on the console; this makes the skin entry point. A second cursor is placed in the lesion to be biopsied. The computer is asked to measure the distance between these two points (i.e. the depth of the lesion from the skin), and also the angle of the path from the vertical.
5. The skin is sterilized, draped and infiltrated with local anaesthetic at the entry site.

6. The biopsy needle is advanced down to the lesion, along the predetermined track, using a ruler to measure the depth and a protractor the angle from vertical.
7. A final scan is taken to check that the needle tip is in the lesion before the biopsy is taken.

How to take the biopsy

1. With the Greene aspiration system, suction is applied by an attached empty syringe. The suction is combined with a rotating motion and cells will be sucked into the needle tip. These cells are immediately smeared on glass slides and fixed in 95% alcohol. Alternatively, cells may be aspirated into a syringe containing a balanced electrolyte solution, to be delivered to the cytopathologist the same day. The fluid can be centrifuged to yield a greater number of cells.
2. If the Rotex screw needle is used, the sheath needle with its trocar are first advanced so that the tip abuts the edge of the lesion. The trocar is removed and is replaced by the screw ended needle. This screw is advanced into the lesion for about 1 cm while the sheath needle remains stationary. Once the core has been fixed on the screw, the screw needle is held stationary while the sheath needle is advanced over it. This cuts off a core around the screw and the whole assemblage is now withdrawn. Material on the screw is immediately plated onto glass slides and fixed in 95% alcohol.
3. The Tru-cut cutting needle should be thoroughly studied before use. A practice biopsy should be taken in air to familiarize oneself with the needle's operation. Once inside the body this large bore needle can do great damage to tissues if the patient breathes. The biopsy must be taken quickly and smoothly, therefore. The needle is advanced into the tissue closed. It is opened by pulling back the outer sheath; tissue prolapses into the receiving slot, the core is cut off by advancing the outer sheath over the stationary inner core and the whole assemblage is removed. The tissue core is usually placed in formalin for histological study.

Post biopsy care

All lung biopsy cases require a post-procedure expiration chest film to identify any pneumothorax.

CHOICE OF BIOPSY NEEDLE

Cutting needles

Cutting needles are usually of large bore with a slotting device to provide a tissue core suitable for histologic sectioning. They should be reserved for large, easily accessible lesions. Large bore needle perforation of bowel, major vessels or the gallbladder is very dangerous and must be avoided. It is wise to anticipate the bleeding risk in patients undergoing large bore needle biopsies by blood typing and cross-matching prior to the procedure.

True aspiration needles

True aspiration needles are variants of the Chiba University needle. These are simple bevelled needles of narrow gauge, which obtain a cytological specimen. The original Chiba needle is of 22 or 23G, very flexible and thus hard to control. The Cook Company market a 21G Chiba variant needle which is less flexible and therefore easier to control. Chiba needles have a 25° bevel. Aspiration needles depend for their action on the negative pressure at their tip created by suction on a syringe at the hub. While suction is applied, the needle tip is moved gently back and forth in the mass. The suction is released and the whole assemblage, with aspirated cells in the needle is removed. The cells are expressed onto glass slides which are then immersed in 95% alcohol.

Modified aspiration needles

Modified aspiration needles are an intermediate group which all provide cells for cytological study, but also very often yield pieces of tissues suitable for histology. The Turner needle (Cook) available in 16, 18, 20 and 22 gauge has a 45° bevel while the Greene needle (Cook) has a square 90° bevel and is available from 18 to 22 gauge. Both of these needles have inner stylettes and are capable of yielding tissue cores. The Rotex (Surgimed) and Franseen (Cook) needles are technically cutting needles; the Rotex of 21 gauge and the Franseen 16, 18, 20 and 22 gauge. However, as they are of narrow calibre, their risks of complication are equivalent to those of aspiration needles. Both are capable of yielding tissue fragments.

ULTRASOUND GUIDED PERCUTANEOUS BIOPSIES AND ASPIRATIONS

Indications

The organs most amenable to this approach are the kidney, liver, pancreas, urinary bladder, abdominal fluid collection, the pregnant uterus, the pericardium, pleura and thyroid.

Equipment

1. A specialized puncture transducer is widely available. This has a central canal through which the biopsy needle is introduced. The needle will follow the direction of the sound beam.

2. For use in the liver and kidney, large needles such as the Menghini or Vim-Silverman types will produce large tissue specimens for histologic examination. These needles may be introduced directly through the puncture transducer.
3. For aspiration of solid abdominal masses, a finer needle such as the Greene 22G is used. When using such a thin needle an outer guide needle may be introduced first to give stability to the needle and to allow multiple passes. This approach also minimizes the spread to tumour cells.

Technique

1. The lesion suitable for puncture is identified by routine scan. The optimal site and direction for puncture are determined.
2. The skin access point is marked on the skin, sterilized and infiltrated with local anaesthetic.
3. The skin is covered with sterile oil and the biopsy transducer, previously sterilized in antiseptic solution is mounted on the scanning arm.
4. The biopsy transducer is placed on the skin and angulated until the sound beam corresponds to the desired access route. The depth of the lesion from the skin is measured. The depth measured, the length of the puncture transducer is marked off on the biopsy needle with a ruler. The biopsy needle is then passed through the transducer by the desired depth down to the lesion.

How to take the biopsy

When the needle is at the desired point in the lesion, a 10 ml syringe is attached. While the needle tip is inside the lesion the syringe plunger is pulled back creating a negative pressure in the system. At the same time the needle tip is moved back and forth three or four times. The negative pressure is released and the needle withdrawn. The cells retrieved are expelled onto glass slides and fixed in 95% alcohol for cytological study.

Hazards

1. Great care must be taken not to pass the needle through major structures especially bowel. The stomach may be traversed by a 21G needle during a pancreatic biopsy however.
2. There is a possible risk of spreading malignant cells along the biopsy route. Such cases have been reported in the literature but overall the risk appears to be low.
3. Subcutaneous haematoma is an occasional occurrence but is unlikely to create a major problem.

SINOGRAPHY AND FISTULOGRAPHY

Indications

Sinograms are usually performed to determine the size, direction and extent of sinuses. Serial studies may be needed to monitor healing. Fistulograms are performed in order to identify the precise anatomy of communications with internal organs and other structures.

Contraindications

1. Heavy wound infection in the presence of fever may lead to septicaemia with manipulation of some sinuses.
2. Infection of wounds with antibiotic resistant organisms may contaminate a procedures' room and make it unusable until thoroughly cleaned. These cases should be done at the end of a list.

Preparation

It is most important that the examiner start the procedure with a complete understanding of the clinical problem and more particularly what information is expected from the examination. The difficulties in sinography become apparent when the examiner is faced with several skin openings of sinus tracks or several external drainage tubes, without a clear understanding of where they lead. For this reason it is essential to have discussed the case with the managing clinician.

Patient sedation, premedication or fasting is usually unnecessary.

Contrast media

A satisfactory general purpose contrast for sinography is meglumine sodium diatrizoate (e.g. Urografin 76%). This water soluble contrast is quickly absorbed by the soft tissues and is generally painless, although may cause pain in the peritoneal cavity. Water soluble contrast should not be used if there is any suggestion of communication with the bronchial tree. If there is such a suspicion, bronchographic contrast medium such as propyliodone (Dionosil) should be used.

Equipment

Some form of introducer is needed to perform a sinogram. Where the orifice is very small a sialogram catheter is best. For larger sinuses a fine soft rubber catheter up to 12 gauge should be used. This may be advanced some distance down the sinus track. For wide-mouthed sinuses, a balloon catheter is very useful. The balloon is inflated and the tip of the catheter introduced into the mouth of the sinus. The patient or an assistant then presses the balloon down onto the skin making an effective seal. Latex and rubber catheters will usually require an 'acorn' adaptor to fit the contrast syringe.

Technique

Initial plain films of the area should be obtained, in order to identify opaque foreign bodies and the position of any existing drain tubes. All films taken during the procedure are best obtained by spot filming at fluoroscopy. This is to allow optimal patient positioning and film centring given that sinuses may run in unexpected directions; also to identify quickly communication with the bowel.

All removable dressings should be taken off and the sinus opening gently cleansed to remove any secretions or crust. The patient is positioned on the fluoroscopic table with the sinus opening uppermost in order to minimize contrast spillage. The sinus is gently probed to determine its principal direction and the catheter, previously filled with contrast and free of bubbles, is introduced. Contrast is injected until it spills back, resistance is felt or the patient complains of pain.

The skin opening of the sinus is marked with an opaque letter, and at least two films, at right angles to each other, are obtained. Oblique films may be necessary to identify fistulous communications with internal organs, or with bone.

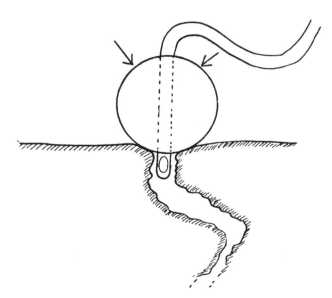

Fig. 7.3 A useful method of introducing contrast into a wide mouthed sinus. The catheter balloon is pressed by the patient or an assistant against the orifice to prevent spillage.

Pitfalls

1. It may not be possible to completely fill very large cavities. In this case the patient should be rotated to different positions with up to 100 ml of contrast injected, in order to determine the extent of the cavity as the contrast moves around the walls. This manoeuvre will avoid missing side channels of the main cavity.
2. If serial examinations are likely to be performed (e.g. over several weeks) it is important that on each occasion the radiologist record in the report, the precise dimensions of the cavity. In this way progress can be easily assessed.
3. Injection pressure of contrast should be gentle in order to minimize the risk of creating false passages or worse, a septicaemia.

BONE BIOPSY

Equipment

The Ackermann biopsy needle set can be used for biopsy of vertebral bodies, sternum, pelvis, extremities and bones of the face and skull. Two sets with different needle lengths are available. The size of the second longer set is indicated in brackets below and the sets contain (Fig. 7.4):
1. 12G skin perforator 4.5 cm long.
2. 12G needle guide cannula 6.5 cm (14 cm) long with a 14G stylette 9.5 cm (17 cm) long. The stylette extends 1 cm beyond needle guide when fitted.
3. 14G short needle 9.7 cm (17.2 cm) long with an obturator 14.5 cm (22 cm) long.

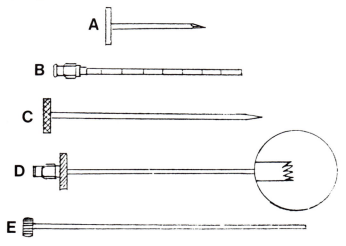

Fig. 7.4 The Ackermann bone biopsy set comprising (A) skin perforator, (B) needle guide cannula, (C) stylette for guide cannula, (D) cutting biopsy needle, (E) obturator for biopsy needle.

4. 14G long needle 11 cm (18.5 cm) long with an obturator 14.5 cm (22 cm) long.

The short needle has six sharp points and extends 1.25 cm beyond the guide. The long needle has six sharp points and extends 2.5 cm beyond the guide.

Preparation

1. Since this procedure is painful, some operators prefer general anaesthesia. This author however uses only an intravenous cocktail of valium 20 mg and pethidine 100 mg, each diluted separately in 10 ml of saline. The mixture is titrated into the patient throughout the procedure to make him oblivious of pain.
2. Local anaesthesia, both in the skin and down to the periosteum is also required.

Technique for thoracic and lumbar vertebral biopsy

1. The patient lies prone on a fluoroscopy table. The back is sterilized and draped.
2. It is essential to have either biplane screening or the facility to take cross table horizontal beam lateral films.
3. The vertebral body to be biopsied is identified and its midline surface marking noted.
4. A point, one hand's breadth to the right of the midline is infiltrated with local anaesthetic. Through this point a 22G spinal needle is passed, angled at 45° from vertical toward the midline, down to the side of the body, infiltrating with local anaesthetic all the way.
5. The position of this needle used as a guide, is checked in two planes at right angles, and any adjustment made. The approach will usually be below the corresponding rib.
6. An adequate skin hole is made at the entry site and the long needle guide cannula with its stylette are advanced down the predetermined track, to the side of the vertebral body.
7. The guide cannula and stylette are tapped with a sterile rubber hammer about 1 cm into the bone cortex to secure the cannula. The stylette is removed.
8. The biopsy needle is advanced through the guide cannula to the bone and screwed into it. The teeth on the tip will cut off a tissue cone which will be held inside the needle.
9. The biopsy needle is withdrawn (leaving the guide cannula). The specimen is pushed out of the needle by the obturator and placed in formalin.
10. The procedure may be repeated if necessary otherwise the guide cannula is also removed.

Difficulties

1. The needle lies too far forward on the side of the vertebral body. The usual cause for this is that the entry point selected is not lateral enough. It is important to approach the side of the vertebral body more en face than tangentially in order to allow the needle guide stylette to bite in.
2. No specimen can be retrieved. If the biopsy needle has been screwed in far enough, the specimen is not being held inside the needle. Two manoeuvres are helpful here. Firstly, an attempt should be made to rock the needle gently back and forth to break off the specimen from its attachment. Secondly, one can apply suction to the needle as it is withdrawn, by means of a syringe, to hold the specimen inside.
3. If all else fails, saline can be flushed down the guide cannula and then aspirated in an attempt to obtain malignant cells for cytological study.

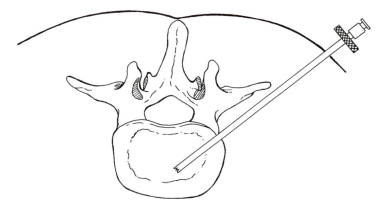

Fig. 7.5 The direction of approach and the final position of an Ackermann biopsy needle inside a lumbar vertebral body.

Cervical vertebral body biopsy

This is a hazardous procedure percutaneously and should only be attempted by an experienced interventional radiologist.

Technique

This is as for other vertebral biopsies except that the patient lies supine and the approach is between the carotid artery laterally and the trachea and oesophagus medially (as in cervical discography).

Bone biopsy elsewhere

Technique

Since most other biopsies are in less hazardous sites than the spine, an appropriate modification of the spinal technique can be applied. The lesion to be biopsied is approached from an entry point vertically above it.

BRONCHOGRAPHY

Indications

The availability of the flexible fibreoptic bronchoscope has reduced the number of indications considerably. The principal ones remaining are:
1. To demonstrate the extent of bronchiectasis.
2. In obscure cases of haemoptysis.
3. To demonstrate bronchial obstruction when bronchoscopy is unavailable or unsuccessful.

Contraindications

1. Allergic reaction to intrabronchial contrast is most unusual and asthma is not a contraindication.
2. Patients with severely limited respiratory reserve should be examined with great caution. In such cases it is often wiser to examine each lung on separate days.

Equipment

The contrast medium can be delivered either via a transnasal catheter passed through the larynx, or by transcricoid needle puncture of the trachea. The transnasal route is preferred as it allows selective filling of the bronchial tree.
1. Jacques and Tiemens catheters 14–18F size.
2. Contrast medium: Aqueous Dionosil (Glaxo).
3. Local anaesthetic spray for the nasopharynx, e.g. Xylocaine 10%.
4. Metal spatula.

Contrast media

The widely used contrast medium Dionosil (propyliodone) is most satisfactory. It is available either as a 50% aqueous suspension or a 60% suspension in arachis oil. The author prefers the aqueous medium since it is his impression that it coats the main bronchi well but does not disperse into the alveoli, a tendency which the oil based medium has. The bottle should be well shaken and warmed in hot water before use. This makes the contrast flow much more readily. If more peripheral filling of the lung is required, Dionosil aqueous may be diluted by adding 1 ml of water to 20 ml of contrast. An average 15 ml of Dionosil is required for each lung.

Patient preparation

1. Nil orally for 4 hours prior to examination.
2. Tuinal or similar barbiturate 100 mg, at 45 minutes prior to procedure and atropine 0.6 mg IM 30 minutes before to suppress the coughing reflex and dry bronchial secretions in order to attain better mucosal coating.

Technique

1. With the patient sitting on the side of an X-ray table the pharynx and larynx are sprayed with local anaesthesia and the nasal cavity on the side with the better airway also.
2. The selected catheter, smeared with Xylocaine jelly, is passed through the nasal cavity until it is seen in the oro pharynx through the mouth. Further local anaesthetic is sprayed into the pharynx whilst the patient takes several deep breaths. Adequate anaesthesia is obtained when the patient stops coughing or gagging each time the spray is applied. Particular attention should be paid to this step since without good local anaesthesia, laryngeal intubation will fail.
3. The patient is warned that as the tube is advanced down the 'windpipe', there will be a strong desire to cough and that this must be resisted, otherwise the tube may be coughed out. The author has found it very useful to talk almost constantly to the patient in a smoothing and encouraging manner throughout the length of this rather unpleasant examination.
4. The patient is asked to hold his tongue forward using a piece of gauze. The head and chin are protruded in a manner similar to that adopted during shaving in a mirror.
5. The patient then breathes rather deeply and during an inspiration the transnasal catheter is advanced rapidly. Successful passage of the tube is usually accompanied by coughing. Xylocaine anaesthetic is then injected down the catheter to anaesthetize the bronchial tree with the patient posturing in various positions.
6. The intratracheal position of the tube may be checked by having the patient exhale, for example, by saying his name, while the end of the tube is submerged in a cup of water. Bubbles will appear from the end of the tube. The ideal position for the tube tip is the mid-trachea.

Contrast installation

The patient is seated on the side of a fluoroscopic table and the right lung is examined first. The lower and middle lobes are filled with Dionosil as the patient leans toward the side being examined, first forward and then backward. In each position the patient is supported by an assistant. The patient then lies on the right side as the upper lobe is filled. Each lung requires approximately 15 ml of contrast. When adequate lobar filling has been checked fluoroscopically, AP, lateral steep and shallow obliques of the right lung with the left side of the chest raised are taken. The procedure is then repeated on the left side, each lobe being filled in turn as the patient leans to the left. The films taken of the left lung are AP steep and shallow oblique with the right side of the chest raised.

Difficulties and complications

1. Failure to pass the catheter. This is usually due to inadequate local anaesthesia. A curved catheter can be used with a spatula to direct local anaesthetic directly to the vocal cords.

2. Coughing. Local anaesthesia is rapidly absorbed from the bronchial mucosa hence the importance of speed. Atropine is important in reducing mucous secretion.

3. Aspiration of food. It is essential that the patient be starved prior to the examination and also for 4 hours after.

Handy hints

If there is persistent difficulty in passing the tube through the vocal cords the following manoeuvres may be attempted.
1. Have the patient rotate the head from side to side while attempting to advance the tube.
2. Make sure that the chin is well forward. This prevents swallowing and tends to direct the tube anteriorly into the larynx.
3. Allow the patient to cough, the tube may slip through the cords during the prolonged inspiration following the cough.
4. Try a tube with pronounced ventral curve or stiffen and curve the tube by inserting a curved guidewire into it.
5. If all else fails the tube may be introduced through the mouth and over the back of the epiglottis by being passed off a 'J' curved wire the tip of which will point the catheter between the cords.

The **right lung** branches are:

1. Apical	)	
2. Anterior	)	Upper lobe
3. Posterior	)	
4. Medial	)	Middle
5. Lateral	)	lobe
6. Apical	)	
7. Medial basal	)	Lower
8. Posterior basal	)	lobe
9. Lateral basal	)	
10. Anterior basal	)	

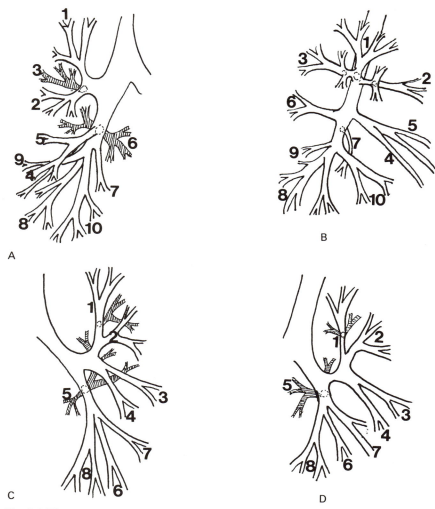

Fig. 7.6 The segmental anatomy of the bronchial tree in the projections used for bronchography, **right** lung in the frontal (A), and lateral (B) positions. **Left** lung in the frontal (C) and left posterior oblique (D) positions.

The **left lung** branches are:
1. Apico-posterior   )
2. Anterior   )   Upper
3. Superior lingular)   lobe
4. Inferior lingular   )
5. Apical   )
6. Posterior basal   )   Lower
7. Lateral basal   )   lobe
8. Anterior basal   )

LARYNGOGRAPHY

Indications

The procedure is usually performed to define the extent of a tumour particularly in a subglottic direction, and to establish the mobility of the vocal cords.

Preparation

The patient should be premedicated with atropine 0.6 mg and a barbituate such as Amylobarbitone 100 mg, 45 minutes before the procedure. These are to dry the laryngeal secretions for better contrast coating and to suppress the coughing reflex respectively. There is usually no need for the patient to fast before the study.

Contrast medium

A suitable medium is Aqueous Dionosil (Propyliodone). Allergic reactions to this are most unusual and asthma is not a contraindication to its use.

Technique

The oropharynx and larngopharynx are anaesthetized with 10% Xylocaine spray. Adequate anaesthesia has been obtained when the patient fails to cough or gag when the throat is sprayed. Particular attention should be paid to spraying the back of the epiglottis and over the vocal cords. A soft rubber catheter such as a 24 French Jacques, lubricated with Xylocaine jelly, is passed through one nostril and advanced down until the tip lies at the back of the epiglottis (Fig. 7.7). The patient stands against an erect fluoroscopy table and by screening in the lateral projection the tube position is checked. Fifteen ml of Dionosil are loaded into a syringe which will require a nozzle adaptor to fit the rubber catheter. With the patient leaning forward and the chin extended, contrast is dripped onto and through the vocal cords, until adequate coating is obtained. The patient should be instructed to cough once or twice to spray the contrast around below the vocal cords.

The following films are taken:
1. One lateral view of the larynx in suspended respiration.
2. Three AP films, one in quiet breathing, one during a Valsalva manoeuvre to appose the cords and one while making the sound 'E' in order to show that the cords move apart.

After the procedure the patient should fast for 4 hours to avoid the risk of aspiration through the anaesthetic larynx.

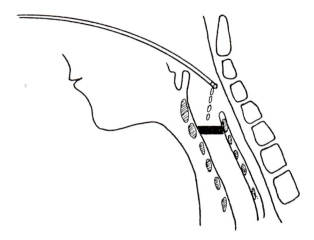

Fig. 7.7 Catheter position to drip contrast onto the vocal cords during laryngography.

NASOPHARYNGOGRAPHY

Indications

This procedure is usually to identify and define the luminal extent of tumour masses.

Preparation

No fasting is necessary. The patient may be premedicated with Amylobarbitone 100 mg 45 minutes before the procedure.

Contrast media

The most satisfactory is bronchographic contrast such as Dionosil (Propyliodone).

Technique

The patient's nasopharynx is anaesthetized by spraying 10% Xylocaine into the nostrils while inhaling deeply. A fine soft rubber tube, such as a 14 French Jacques, lubricated with Xylocaine jelly, is inserted along the floor of one nostril for a short distance. The patient lies supine on a radiographic table with the shoulders elevated on a pillow and the head well extended. Ten ml of Dionosil are instilled into the nasopharynx. The following well penetrated films are now taken; a single base view of the skull with the head extended, a right and left lateral view of the nasopharynx with the patient lying on the side and using a vertical X-ray beam. In this way the roof, posterior and lateral walls of the nasopharynx will be visualized.

DACROCYSTOGRAPHY

Indications

The most usual reason for this procedure is a weeping eye and the most usual cause of the condition is obstruction of the lacrimal passages, at the level of the lacrimal punctum, the nasal cavity or in the ducts between these two.

Contraindications

Acute infections of the eye.

Anatomy of the normal lacrimal system

There are upper and lower lacrimal puncta on the medial end of the upper and lower eyelid. From each of these, a lacrimal canaliculus drains to the ampulla from which tears flow through mucosal valves of Rosenmuller into the lacrimal sac. This structure is approximately 1 cm long and lies on the lateral side of the nasal bone. From its distal end; the valve of Krause opens into naso-lacrimal duct which traverses two other valves, of Taillefer and Hasner, to open into the nasal cavity below the inferior nasal turbinate bone.

Special points of note are:
1. The puncta are only visible when the eyelids are everted.
2. The lower canaliculus has a vertical and horizontal component (see Fig. 7.7).

Preparation

No local anaesthesia is usually necessary. In fact if anaesthesis is used the patient will require an eye pad at the end of the procedure to protect the cornea against foreign body damage. The procedure is performed on an outpatient basis and no premedication is required.

Radiography

A magnification technique is highly desirable. This is achieved by simply increasing the patient–film distance. The films taken are a true lateral of the duct and a 30° mento-occipital view. These may be taken with the patient supine, or if no magnification is to be used, the patient may sit erect against a vertical film holder. The former is preferred.

Technique

The patient lies supine on the radiographic table. Any fluid in the lacrimal sac is expressed by pressing on the side of the nose. The patient is instructed to look upward and outward and the inferior punctum is displayed by everting the lower eyelid. The punctum is gently dilated with a Nettleship dilator and a blunt lacrimal cannula previously filled with contrast and with gas bubbles excluded is advanced into the lacrimal canaliculus. The ideal contrast medium is either Endografin 50%, an aqueous solution of the methyl glucamine salt of tri-olo benzoic acid or Lipiodol (iodized ethyl ester of poppy seed oil).

Contrast medium is injected either until it is tasted by the patient in the mouth or until it refluxes out of the superior lacrimal punctum. Usually 1–2 ml of contrast is required. Lateral and 30° mento-occipital films are then taken.

Problems

1. If the inferior lacrimal duct appears to be occluded, the procedure may be repeated via the superior punctum.
2. Great care must be taken not to rupture the canaliculi. This can be avoided by using only blunt instruments, directing the lacrimal cannula medially after a short vertical course (i.e. appreciating the vertical and horizontal components of the lacrimal canaliculus) and gentle technique particularly with the dilator.
3. Cannulation of the lacrimal canaliculus may be found easier if a Rabinov type sialogram extension catheter is used.

Dacrocystogram equipment

Sialogram pack

1. One kidney dish.
2. Two small lotion bowls.
3. One blunt drawing up needle.
4. One nettleship dilator (blunt).
5. Two lacrymal probes.
6. Two blunt lacrymal needles 23G.
7. Gauze swabs.
8. Contrast – Endografin.
9. Rabinov sialogram catheters size 16 and 32.
10. Disposable syringes 2 ml and 10 ml.
11. Bright light.

SIALOGRAPHY

Indications

1. Recurrent salivary gland swelling.
2. To demonstrate sialectasis.

3. To demonstrate salivary duct obstruction.
4. To localize a palpable salivary gland tumour.

Equipment

1. Punctum dilator.
2. Rabinov disposable sialography needle sets — small and large size.
3. Concentrated water soluble contrast medium, e.g. Endografin.
4. A slice of lemon, a wooden spatula, and a torch.

Patient preparation

Gauze soaked in local anaesthetic is applied to the duct orifice.

Technique

1. An initial set of plain films are taken. For the parotid gland they are an AP (tangential to the gland) and transpharyngeal lateral oblique. For the submandibular gland a supero-inferior intra-oral film and a transpharyngeal lateral oblique are taken to identify duct calculi.
2. The duct orifice is dilated with the punctum dilator.
3. The blunt end of the Rabinov needle is introduced into the duct, the needle and tubing having been filled with contrast medium beforehand.
4. The patient gently closes the mouth on the tubing during filming.
5. Only a very small amount, approximately 1 ml should be injected.

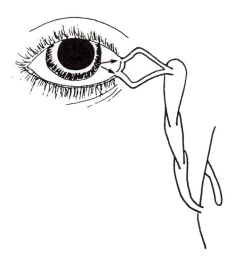

Fig. 7.8 Anatomy of the lacrimal duct system. Arrows point to the superior and inferior lacrimal canaliculi.

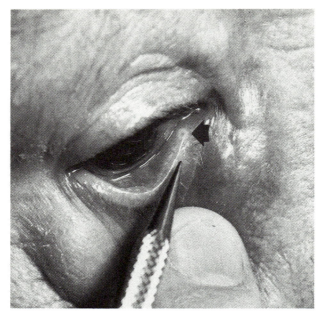

Fig. 7.9 The inferior lacrimal punctum (arrow) exposed by everting the lower eyelid.

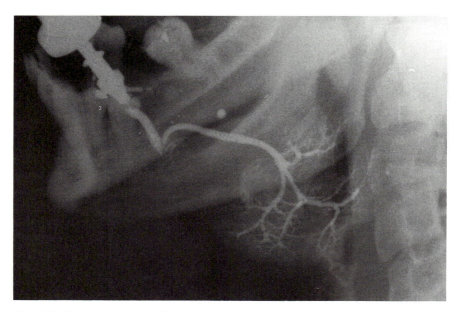

Fig. 7.10 The normal submandibular sialogram.

Instead of a syringe the Rabinov tubing can be elevated to allow filling by gravity.

6. Contrast films are taken in the same projection as the plain films.

Difficulties and complications

1. Difficulty in identifying the duct orifice. The pathological gland frequently produces less saliva. Stimulation of secretion with a slice of lemon may assist in identifying the ostium.
2. Overfilling. A spurious appearance suggesting sialectasis can be produced by overfilling. The appearance is due to contrast passing through the duct lining to lie in the periductal tissue.

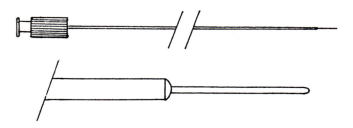

Fig. 7.11 The Rabinov sialography tube with a magnified view of the blunt distal metal needle. The tubing length is 32 cm, and the tip diameter ranges from small (primarily for submandibular ducts) to large (primarily for parotid ducts or intravenous cholangiography).

BREAST LUMP NEEDLE LOCALIZATION

Indications

To fix the position of an impalpable breast mass prior to surgical biopsy.

Equipment

The disposable Kopans type localization needle is a 21G needle containing a hook tipped wire, with such an arrangement that when the tip of the wire is advanced out of the needle tip, the hook opens and secures it in the breast tissue (Fig. 7.12).

Technique

1. An initial mammogram is performed with supero-inferior and lateral views.
2. The distance of the mass from the nipple is measured on both the above views and a suitable entry point marked on the skin.

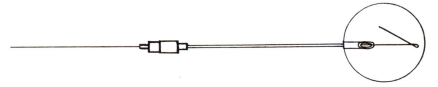

Fig. 7.12 The Kopans type breast localization needle. The needle is advanced into position with the wire hook closed inside it. When the inner wire is advanced the hook springs open and anchors itself in the tissues.

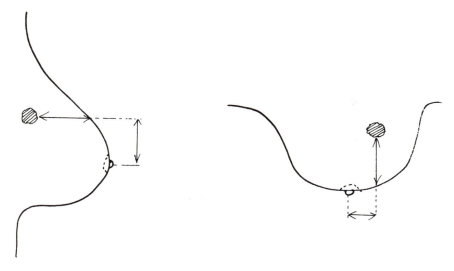

Fig. 7.13 The optimal entry point for the breast localization needle and the depth of the lump from the surface are estimated from the preliminary lateral and supero-inferior films.

3. The entry point is cleansed and the skin infiltrated with local anaesthetic.
4. The Kopans needle with the hook closed inside is advanced to the predetermined depth and at an angle judged to be correct.
5. A single film, supero-inferior or lateral is taken and an appropriate adjustment to the needle position made.
6. If the needle position is satisfactory in one plane, the plane at right angles is taken and if again acceptable the·hook is released from the needle tip and the external wire taped to the patient's skin.

HYSTERO-SALPINGOGRAPHY

Indications

1. To show the shape and position of the uterine body.

2. To demonstrate the patency or otherwise of the fallopian tubes, thus possible causes of infertility.
3. To show congenital anomalies such as biconuate uterus.
4. To show masses such as intraluminal polyps or intra-uterine adhesions as in Asherman's syndrome.

Contraindications

1. Pregnancy.
2. Suspected ectopic pregnancy because of the danger of tubal rupture.
3. Acute infection of the vagina or cervix because of the danger of dissemination of infection.
4. The week prior to menstruation. At this time the endometrium is thick and vascular. There is a greater than usual danger of venous lymphatic injection of contrast, particularly if oily medium is used.
5. The week following menstruation. The endometrium has been substantially lost and there is a similar danger of contrast injection as in 4.

Contrast media

The two available groups of contrast are oily and aqueous. Each has advantages and disadvantages.

Water soluble media

There are several of these media available and they are equally good. The principal ones are:
(a) Endografin (50% aqueous solution of the methyl glucamine salt of tri-iodobenzoic acid).
(b) Diaginol viscous (40% solution of sodium acetrizoate with dextran).
(c) Urographin 76% (sodium and methylglucamine salts of tri-iodobenzoic acid).

Water soluble contrast media flow more easily than oily media and so peritoneal spill is more readily seen. They are more irritant to the peritoneum than oily media but have the very great advantage of not causing a significant problem if accidental intravenous injection occurs.

Oily media

The principal oily medium is Lipiodol (iodized ethyl ester of poppy seed oil). This has the advantage of causing little discomfort in the peritoneal cavity and provides good mucosal coating. However, it flows less readily than aqueous media and so peritoneal spill may be considerably delayed. There is the ever present danger of oil embolism, should the contrast find its way intravenously. For these reasons, the author prefers to use aqueous contrast such as Endografin, which will give very good results.

Preparation

1. The patient should be premedicated with 10 mg Valium IM or IV.
2. No fasting is necessary.

Technique

The patient is placed in the lithotomy position on a fluoroscopic table. The vulva is sterilized and the perineum and legs are draped in sterile fashion. A 'duckbill' speculum is inserted into the vagina and the cervix is visualized. The cap of the suction tube is applied to the cervix with the inner tube in the cervical canal (Fig. 7.14). Suction is applied to the cup with the attached pump. Contrast is now slowly injected until peritoneal spill is noted from either fallopian tube. A single AP film of the pelvis is sometimes sufficient if contrast spills from both tubes. Right and left oblique or a 10-minute delayed film may be necessary. In most cases it is useful to apply mild downward traction on the cervix in order to unfold the usual anteversion of the uterus (Fig. 7.15).

Difficulties

1. Inability to visualize the cervix can be overcome by bimanual palpation to establish its position and then widely opening the speculum blades in that region.

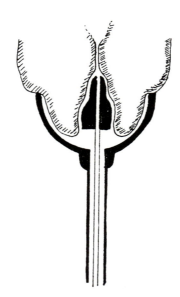

Fig. 7.14 The arrangement of the Malmström–Westman suction cannula in the cervical canal. The outer suction cup holds the exterior of the cervix while the inner catheter with a conical tip lies in the opening of the cervical canal.

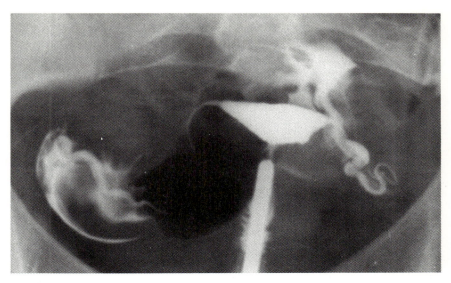

Fig. 7.15 A normal hystero-salpinogram, showing patent fallopian tubes demonstrated by the bilateral contrast spill into the peritoneal cavity.

2. Inability to create suction on the cervix is usually due to the cup being too large. Select one of a size more appropriate to the cervix.

PNEUMOPERITONEUM

Indications

This is a rarely performed procedure, but the author is called upon to perform one per year by thoracic surgeons as treatment for recurrent and persistent pneumothorax. It may also be used to diagnose a peritoneal–pleural fistula by producing a pneumothorax.

Technique

With the patient supine on a fluoroscopic table, a point midway between the umbilicus and the symphysis pubis is selected, sterilized and infiltrated with local anaesthetic. A 22G short bevel spinal needle is passed through the entry point and angled toward the head. As it is passed deeper, a sudden pressure and release is felt as the needle passes through the peritoneum. At this point the patient will feel a sudden sharp pain. A small amount (5 ml) of room air is injected. This should pass without resistance into the peritoneal cavity and fluoroscopy will show that no air is collected around the needle tip.

For a therapeutic pneumoperitoneum, 2–3 l of room air are injected. Before injecting any air, it is most important to draw back on the syringe to ensure that the needle tip is not in a vessel. If all goes as it should, the patient will notice shoulder tip pain and gas will be visible under the diaphragm when the table is tipped 45° upright. The air can be expected to remain in the peritoneal cavity for 24–48 hours.

REFERENCES

Gerzof S G, Spira R, Robbins A H 1981 Percutaneous abscess drainage. Seminars in Roentgenology 16: 62–71

Martin E C, Harison K B, Fankuchen E I, Cooperman A, Casarella W J 1982 Percutaneous drainage of postoperative intraabdominal abscesses. American Journal of Roentgenology 138: 13–15

Van Sonnenberg E, Ferrucci J T, Mueller P R 1982 Percutaneous drainage of abscesses and fluid collections. Tehnique results and applications. Radiology 142: 1–10

FURTHER READING

Ackermann W 1956 Vertebral trephine biopsy. Annals of Surgery 143: 373–385

Ackermann W 1963 Application of the trephine for bone biopsy: results of 635 cases. Journal of the American Medical Association 184: 11–17

Avnet N L, Elkin M 1967 Hysterosalpingography. Radiologic Clinics of North America 5 (No 1) 105–120

Campbell W 1964 The radiology of the lacrimal system. British Journal of Radiology 37: 1–26

de Santos L A, Lukeman J M, Wallace S, Murray J A, Alaya A G 1978 Percutaneous needle biopsy of bone in the cancer patient. American Journal of Roentgenology 130: 641–649

Dunnick N R, Fisher R I, Chu E W 1980 Percutaneous aspiration of retroperitoneal lymph nodes in ovarian cancer. American Journal of Roentgenology 135: 109–113

Ferrucci J T Jr, Wittenberg J 1978 CT biopsy of abdominal tumours: aide for lesion localization. Radiology 129: 739–744

Ferrucci J T Jr, Wittenberg J, Mueller P R et al 1980 Diagnosis of abdominal malignancy by radiologic fine needle biopsy. American Journal of Roentgenology 134: 323–330

Haaga J R, Vanek J 1979 Computed tomographic guided liver biopsy using the Menghini needle. Radiology 133: 405–408

Isler R J, Ferrucci J T, Wittenberg J et al 1981 Tissue core biopsy of abdominal tumours with a 22 gauge cutting needle. American Journal of Roentgenology 136: 725–728

Kopans D B, DeLuca S 1980 A modified needle-hookwire technique to simplify preoperative localization of occult breast lesions. Radiology 134:781

Liebermann R P, Hafez G R, Crummy A B 1982 Histology from aspiration biopsy: Turner needle experience. American Journal Roentgenology 138: 561–564

Lumsden K, Truelove S C 1957 Diagnostic pneumoperitoneum. British Journal of Radiology 30: 516

Powers W E, McGee H H, Seaman W B 1957 The contrast examination of larynx and pharynx. Radiology 68: 169–177

Powers W E, Holtz S, Ogura J 1964 Contrast examination of the larynx and pharynx: inspiratory phonation. American Journal of Roentgenology 92: 40–42

Rabinov K R, Joffa N 1969 A blunt tip side injecting cannula for sialography. Radiology 92: 1438

Schwerk W B, Durr H K, Schmitz-Moormann P 1983 Ultrasound guided fine needle biopsies in pancreatic and hepatic neoplasms. Gastrointestinal Radiology 8: 219–225

Yune H Y, Klatte E C 1972 Current status of sialography. American Journal of Roentgenology 115: 420–428

Zavala D C, Schoell J E 1981 Ultrathin Needle Aspiration of the Lung in Infectious and Malignant Disease. American Review of Respiratory Disease 123: 125–131

Index